Problems
IN CHILD BEHAVIOR
AND DEVELOPMENT

Problems

IN CHILD BEHAVIOR
AND DEVELOPMENT

MILTON J. E. SENN, M.D.

Sterling Professor of Pediatrics and Psychiatry, Yale University School of Medicine; Former Director, Yale Child Study Center, New Haven.

ALBERT J. SOLNIT, M.D.

Professor of Pediatrics and Psychiatry, Yale University School of Medicine; Director, Yale Child Study Center, New Haven, Connecticut.

Lea & Febiger   Philadelphia • 1968

To Blanche and Martha

Preface

MANY CHANGES have taken place in pediatric practice during the past three decades. There has been a lowered incidence of many childhood diseases and their complications, brought about by prophylactic measures as well as more specific therapy in treating infections. Concurrently there has been an increase in the numbers of children remaining alive with physical defects and chronic illness. Then too, there have been demands of parents for the physician to become involved in the care of the child when he is well, guidance in child rearing as well as prophylactic measures against the common communicable diseases. Thus there is an imperative need for the physician who practices medicine with child patients actively to help parents and children when there are problems of behavior and development.

Unfortunately, the favorable shifts downward in the frequency of childhood disease have not been paralleled by a decrease in the number of persons who are emotionally disturbed to a degree where they need help from professional persons. Nor has there been an appreciable increase in the number of individuals who by special training and experience could provide the professional assistance so urgently needed. The numerical limitations of psychiatrists, social workers and psychologists is matched by their inaccessibility to people in distress who for one reason or another prefer to get help (at least in the beginning) from non-psychiatric physicians, clergymen and various laymen.

The non-psychiatric physician as a first line of defense has many assets as well as limitations to his functioning adequately as a diagnostician and therapist in the field of emotional disturbances. His medical school training in this area has often been inadequate, even though he graduated from a grade A institution as recently as this year. The physician who has been sensitive over the years to his patients' needs and to his own adequacy to help, inevitably became dissatisfied with himself. He considered ways of furthering his knowledge but usually ended up deciding that self-education is the only realistic approach open to him.

Concurrent with the changes that were taking place in pediatrics, as the biological sciences and other medical disciplines contributed to the improvement of child health and care, significant changes also occurred in the social sciences, particularly those embracing psychology, sociology, psychiatry, psychoanalysis and child development. Orthodoxy has ruled less supremely than heretofore, and eclecticism is now favored by even those persons specifically identified with certain schools of personality theory such as psychoanalysis and learning theory.

Our decision to write another book for pediatricians and general practitioners, despite the ready availability of other good texts, was determined by three major goals. (1) We wanted to encourage pediatricians who as non-psychiatrists have an interest in and a wish to help patients psychologically. (2) As pioneers in teaching non-psychiatric physicians about parental guidance and the management of psychologic disorders in infants and children, it was our wish to describe the philosophy and methods at the Yale Child Study Center of dealing with parents and children in distress. We do not imply that what we do is the best and only way of meeting the situations, but that we have had some measure of success and much pleasure. Then, too, we have been asked repeatedly by our students, pediatric residents, practitioners in general medicine and pediatrics for written material on our way of working. (3) Finally, we hoped to make suggestions of how to use non-medical associates as colleagues, to work in close association with the pediatrician or at some distance.

At the present time, all health professions are confronted with problems of how to deal satisfactorily and helpfully with the many patients in need of their services. This has led to consideration by many professional organizations of the desirability to form new careers, in which lay people after short courses are able to take over some of the care now provided by physicians and other workers. We have not experimented with such training but have often recommended to pediatricians in private practice that they engage as colleagues persons already established in their careers, particularly social workers and clinical psychologists. The concept behind this is that a *team* concerning itself with physical and emotional health may more realistically cope with both sets of problems than a physician alone.

The aim of this book then is to present our methods of approaching problems in child and family behavior, and to update some concepts in child development, psychiatry and psychoanalysis which heretofore have appeared in various pediatric texts. Our desire is to help physicians in practical ways to deal with problems which parents bring to the pediatrician and general practitioner even before the birth of the baby and up to the time of mid-adolescence.

An attempt has been made to keep the arrangement of this book simple. Essays will be kept to a minimum in an effort to avoid replication of material to be found in other books. Although we deal with many topics, we hope not to inundate our readers and thus weaken the impact of those things that we think they really ought to know. Anecdotes and short case histories will be interspersed with the essay materials in the hope that they will illuminate "some dark corners of ignorance." Other case histories, some long and some short, will also be presented to provide the reader with a study of each clinical situation and the diagnosis that will suggest appropriate management. For the most part cases will demonstrate the vicissitudes of development from infancy to adolescence and our basic method of approach to these problems; i.e. to study a child's problems in relation to his stage of development in the family and in the community.

The cumulative, stored knowledge that the pediatrician can acquire about each of his patients and their families enables him to become a medical expert on that child, that family. This book is written with the additional aim of demonstrating how to mitigate the inevitable tendency to fragment medical care as a consequence of the recent explosion of knowledge about children. The pediatrician who can use himself as a healing instrument will develop his relationship with the child and family as a vehicle that will promote the delivery of integrated medical care including referrals for special care when it is indicated. Integrated medical care as we conceive of it includes the promotion of healthy development, the prevention of iatrogenic disorders, and the effective treatment of illness.

The focus in this book is not only on the management of life situations which are full blown, but it also is directed at suggesting preventive measures which in the hands of an insightful physician may ward off problems, or at least make them more amenable to solution. In using the book the physician in a hurry will naturally seek in the index the topic which interests him. Frequent cross-references will guide him to those pages which will help him cope with the problems of the patient which concern him at that time. In a more leisurely period, the physician may be interested to read whole sections of the book, particularly those dealing with theories of personality development.

For brevity, the list of bibliographic references has been restricted to those which seem of particular value to us as practitioners. In acknowledging assistance to other persons in the preparation of this book, few are singled out for special words of gratitude because the number of individuals to whom we are in debt for stimulation, enlightenment and assistance is too long. We are mindful of the help and encouragement received not only from many professional persons, but from innumerable children and their parents as well.

Special gratitude is due to Dr. Sally Provence for her contributions on the section *Predicting Development* (Chapter 8), to Mrs. Claire Hartford for editorial assistance, and Jennie Parthenios for meticulous and painstaking secretarial help.

MILTON J. E. SENN
ALBERT J. SOLNIT

New Haven, Connecticut

Contents

Chapter 1

INTRODUCTION AND THEORETICAL CONSIDERATIONS

Basic Concepts Regarding Personality Development

Several important theories have evolved about the personality development of infants and children. The most popular today are those stemming from Freudian psychoanalytic theory, particularly that of Erikson on stages of affective development. Equally important are Piaget's concepts of cognitive development, and the learning theories. More recently the field of animal studies (ethology) have provided concepts of the "imprinting" process in development. Unfortunately there is yet no common language in these various, and sometimes conflicting, theories. And certainly none has earned universal acceptance.

With this in mind, our theoretical inclinations are eclectic. In our use of Freudian theory it will be obvious to the sophisticated reader that we do not apply Freudian instinctual theory narrowly. Like Erikson we are mindful of the constant and penetrating influence of the many factors of the environment. We therefore present an applied version of Freudian psychoanalytic principles, and Piaget's concepts of cognitive learning and socialization, only as they apply to our discussion of clinical material. Together these theories have contributed to our concept that personality of the infant and child is the product of progressive development.

This book characterizes the developmental phases as they appear chronologically, and as they evolve qualitatively, in the growing child. But having said this, we also state categorically that these phases are not to be viewed as narrow landmarks, but as broad periods of transition which logically flow from one to the other over time, and through the integration of acquired experiences. Each of these stages have certain dominant characteristics which portray the simultaneous functions of affective and cognitive features that operate within the physical

1

and social milieu. By understanding the expected dynamic flow of development, we can see and evaluate any pathological interruption or interference with them.

We stress that a child develops from an organism characterized by immaturity and irrational behavior to a state when he is master of himself and of his fate, as far as it is possible for him to be. We know generally what the steps are along the way (the phases of development) and we have a general approximation of the times when they are expected to occur. We also know the characteristic symptoms that are manifest or expected in these phases of maturation, and what they presage. The unknown quality, the "x" in the formula, is how the specific child, with his own unique endowment and under the circumstances of his particular environment, will fulfill *his* maturation. This is the crux of many a pediatric problem and it is the subject matter of this book.

Since the pediatrician is already accustomed to considering an individual child's physical development along longitudinal lines, with maturational anlage as well as other intrinsic and extrinsic idiosyncratic factors, it is logical that behavioral aspects should also be viewed in this light.

It is important for the pediatrician, who deals with the problems of diagnosis and treatment and views them developmentally, to be aware that the attitudes and behavior of parents also have developmental sequences which accompany those of the child. They too undergo shifts, changes and variations in their attitudes and behavior, concomitant with those of the child. Through the process of interaction in sequential phases of development, parents and child play a cause-effect role with each other.

This forces one to a study of the family. The family should be considered not only as a sociological and cultural unit, but also as a psychological unit within which the family member under diagnostic scrutiny is identified. A study of the family reveals the way in which the communication of conscious and unconscious aims and wishes is mediated among members of a family group. It discloses also the shifting dominances, alignments and preferences within it, and the relationship of such shifts to developmental changes in the "problem" child. Within the context of the family, one can also fruitfully study the part that the child's relationship with his siblings and other children plays in his development. The family is seen as a unit of growth and experience, as an organic unit in which the action of any member affects the others.

The child's world is also constructed out of other worlds, which makes it imperative that one understand the general culture and the sub-cultures in which children are reared in order to understand them fully. Our discussion of child development therefore cannot be exclusively child oriented. The approaches of Piaget, Gesell and some psychoanalytic schools are almost too exclusively child oriented. But even these recognize the reciprocal pattern of behavior between mother and child as it unfolds from birth onwards. In considering the nature of the child, one invariably must consider the primary roles of his parents, and of those other persons as well, who are of near primary significance in influencing him and hence responsible to some degree for what he is, how he behaves, and what he becomes.

Psychoanalytic theory provides a base for understanding human development. Freudian theory teaches that the child's personality and mental functioning emerge from the continuous dynamic interactions of his instinctual, biologically-based drive forces (id), his dawning self-regulative capacities (ego and superego) and the nurturing, socializing gratifications and demands that characterize his environment. The instinctual drives cannot be observed directly but only as derivatives of psychosocial development and behavior, since the drive forces, sexual and aggressive, are always expressed and discerned in relationship to the child's tolerances and what he discharges or communicates to the care-taking adult, his parent.

Although the infant begins life as a completely self-centered and dependent individual, driven by his id forces, the development of the ego and superego are not slow in coming. Ego development probably begins in a rudimentary fashion at birth, is dependent upon the integrity of the central nervous system and especially on intactness of the perceptual apparatus. The ego is that part of the mind which perceives, thinks, remembers, takes note of the outside world and conceptualizes the self as having a boundary which delineates it from the non-self. This concept of the ego function is useful to the neurologist in analyzing various subjective phenomena of his patients who have distortions of their body image.

Already by the age of 2 and 3 years, the child has an ego which is well along in its development. As it develops it provides him with a sense of difference from other people and other objects, some sense of reality, ability to use his unconscious to develop mechanisms of defense, a competence in cognition and in use of intelligence, and a questioning attitude about fair play. It serves also as a prelude to concern regarding moral and ethical decision-making. While this latter characteristic is at an unsophisticated level, the child does ask about what is bad and good, and he shows the beginning of a superego and conscience. He anticipates and fears punishment because he has displeased those adults whom he loves, and whose loss of love would be catastrophic. These adults are usually his parents after whom he has largely shaped his conscience, using them first as his outer controlling agent and then incorporating their ideals and values into himself by the time he enters primary school. Ultimately, from this comes self control.

In adults, mental health may be viewed as a balance between the instinctual (id) and ego forces, with a minimum amount of discomfort or frustration. Further, we take into consideration the capacity for loving, for working with others, for successful accomplishment of sex and work, and ability to attract more social praise than social condemnation.

But with a child, particularly in his early years, there is a normal proclivity for imbalance, for disequilibrium and for conflict between the instinctual and the developing ego forces. Conflicts are frequent between the developing ego and superego, and the id. The defenses used while appropriate for the child, when measured against adult behavior, would be considered abnormal. In childhood, disequilibrium is normal because conscious, preconscious and unconscious processes are in continuous instability. The child seems more controlled by unconscious forces than by his conscious will. He is dirty, messy, easily given to rage, uninhibited in speech, impulsive, sexually exhibitionistic, particularly auto-erotic, and his sex play with peers infantile.

Psychoanalytic Theory

In a sense the developmental sequences in personality formation depend on what happens to the sex drive and the aggressive drive. But this cannot be divorced from many modifying and moderating influences that include: the intensity and tempo of drive demands; the soothing, gratifying or frustrating reactions and demands of the parents; the child's innate capacities to tolerate drive build-up, to accept substitutes for direct gratification and to divert or channel his impulsive drive forces into a variety of expressions or behavior. The latter functions are the forerunners of what are to become the functions of the ego.

The energy behind the sexual drives of childhood and adulthood is viewed as psychic energy—"the demand the body makes upon the mind" (Freud, 3 Essays). This is a metaphoric way of describing the nature of the psychic energy that is referred to as libido for the sexual drives, and as aggressive energies for the aggressive drives. Instinctual drives are appetitive, originally non-specific in regard to the target of their thrust, and subject to modification. The original modifications result from a combination of the child's tolerances, his reflex and motor characteristics and the ways in which he is gratified and protected from excessive frustrations and stimulation. One, indeed, cannot speak of an infant without speaking of its parents, especially the mother.

Psychoanalysts speak of libidinal phases of the sexual drive beginning with orality (roughly the first year and a half of life), anality (approximately from 12 months through the second birthday), phallic development (approximately after the second birthday through the fifth and sixth years), latency (corresponding to the school years from 5 to 12 years), followed by preadolescence, and then adolescence. There is considerable overlapping of these phases.

Concurrent with the libidinal sex drive is that of the aggressive instinct. Both are assumed to be present at the time of birth. This system of drives constitutes what is called the id. The newborn infant is egocentric, completely dependent, more or less reflex acting. The behavioral characteristics of the infant and the response of the mother to him in this earliest period of mother-child interaction will be described later in discussing the nature of infancy and the succeeding periods of childhood.

Suffice it to say now, that in the first period of orality the mouth is an important instrument not only for the taking in of nourishment, but for the expression of aggressive tendencies through sucking and for the obtaining of pleasure from that and from swallowing. Nearly all available objects brought in contact with the mouth, besides being tested and made familiar, provide pleasurable stimulation. Object-sucking, especially finger-sucking, is a good example of a normal response but one which may cause concern and anxiety to the mother. Attempts to break the habit meet resistance on the part of the baby, proving the strength of this drive and, in the opinion of the mother, of the will of the baby.

From approximately 1 year onward the role of the mouth for need-gratification (in psychoanalytic theory, of an erotogenic nature) is complemented by heightened sensitivity to the skin around the anus. In part, this stems from the attention and abundant stimulation focussed on that region during the long period of toilet training. Not only does a child develop great interest in the whole process of elimination, enjoying the attention to the anal region, but he also derives special pleasure from use of his mouth in biting, spitting and chewing. The preschool child in this period of anality, as it merges into the next phase of phallic development, also shows his aggressive drive in hitting and kicking, destroying objects and throwing temper tantrums.

Sometime about the age of $2\frac{1}{2}$ years, interest begins to be centered on the genital parts of the body, the so-called phallic period. The boy enjoys showing off his penis, engages in urinary play, and the girl expresses envy in being deprived of a penis. She invariably demonstrates some fear of sexual difference at this time, when curiosity about differences between boys and girls, and the nature of intimacy between parents are topics of frank talk by both sexes. Sometimes this is embarrassing and even frightening to parents who worry that their children may be headed for a life of sexual perversion.

The aggressive drive in this period is demonstrated by overbearing, domineering and forceful attitudes. The boy has to demonstrate his masculinity, his strength and his superiority over girls. How much of this is a learned response and how much is based on his masculine sex drive remains a problem for discussion among the specialists in child development. Genital masturbation for the first time reaches a high point now, a prelude to more mature genital activities. Sex play between the sexes and with the same sex at this time may also be considered perverse by some parents, but when viewed from the point of view of adult genitality it may appear precocious. From a developmental point of view, all these manifestations are normal not only when they first appear, but as they persist to some degree through adolescence and adult life.

Adolescence, of course, brings in the usual overt manifestation of sex development, with much autoerotic behavior, and sex activity with children of the same and opposite sex. The adolescent demonstrates his aggressive drive in a variety of ways. Those particularly difficult to comprehend by parents are the inconsiderateness towards others, the anti- and dissocial outbursts, mental cruelty and the ruthless competitiveness. When directed towards the environment, the aggressive forces serve the purpose of self-preservation to some degree but also provide a means of helping the child test himself and the world outside. Viewed this way the behavior is to be considered normal and healthy. When his aggressive tendencies are directed inwards, they threaten his own bodily and mental health, particularly when they lead to ideas of self-destruction and depression.

Thus psychoanalytic theory provides an overall view of human development and behavior. It includes concern for biologic determinants and for interaction with other persons, especially parents, in a particular environment. There is regard for the maturational and developmental aspects of personality formation and for the mechanisms and processes which make for progression or regression, for adaptation or failure to cope. In other words, this theoretical system views the human being as originating from a biologic state endowed with his particular genic heredity and his personal constitution, and evolving through a series of stages or epochs which are shaped by extrinsic influences as well. An end point is reached which may be optimum for that individual or short of his potential, which may be satisfying or not satisfying according to standards set by himself or by others.

Maturation may be regarded as the process of biologic growth which is an inherent capacity of the child and follows a biologic timetable. Although every person develops along the same biologic pathway, the epochs reached, as well as the chronology of their appearance, vary from one individual to another. In part this is due to the different potentials with which each is born, but also because his development is the result of the interaction of intrinsic factors with the environment. There are also causes for difference between people because each person has his own particular family and his private personal world. This accounts for the fact that we are no longer able to view behavior so narrowly as to consider every trait universally held, nor if universal to accept its significance as identical for every society. A trait such as aggression, although universal, does not make its appearance in each person by a specific chronological age, nor does aggression in one culture have the same significance as that in another.

Child development workers no longer talk about the years as the "terrible 2's," the "trusting 3's," or "the fighting 4's." These expressions may have seemed alliteratively apt, but they were scientifically incorrect. Age norms established by Gesell for psychomotor development in infancy continue to have validity. Unfortunately, there are no analogous specifically age related standards of emotional maturation or of behavior. Here age is but one variable along with heredity, constitution, sex, social class, historical and cultural setting which makes behavior what it is, and determines the nature of one's personality.

Progress is best determined by measuring a child against himself from time to time instead of merely comparing him by age and sex against normative standards of height, weight, behavior and personality traits. Taking note of characteristic sequences and viewing behavior in the context in which it appears and in terms of its meaning for *that* child, in that particular time and place in *his* life, tells one much more about a child and his problems.

Uppermost in the minds of parents who are concerned about a child's behavior is whether it is "normal" or not. Such a concern is shared by pediatricians and teachers. Hence some knowledge is necessary of what is "usual" to serve as a baseline for comparing traits which may be deviant. Yet normality is difficult to measure. Statistical evaluation is of little help in deciding whether traits are appropriate for a particular child. Value judgments come into play in assessing behavior even more than in analyzing physical development.

Such commonly used words as adjustment, adaptation, integration, are psychologic terms which one uses in describing a child's reaction to life situations. But their use as measures of normality must carry some sense of the relativity of performance in assessing whether behavior is appropriate or inappropriate.

What may be normal adaptation for one individual may be maladaptation for another; what may be a normal adaptation at one time of life may not be viewed as healthy at another time in the life of that child. When is anxiety about one's performance in school or at work normal or abnormal? Isn't striving for intellectual perfection a "normal" adaptation to the facts of life, and always accompanied by some anxiety? When does anxiety become a psychologic defense mechanism which prevents one from engaging in experiences which are too stressful? These are the type of questions a physician faces in assessing behavior which is brought to him because someone is concerned by it.

Often we set limits arbitrarily as a dividing line between what is normal and abnormal. For example, today pediatricians are not unusually disturbed if a child wets the bed occasionally up to his fifth birthday. But why the fifth birthday? To some parents this age is too late, and others view it as too early. When the date concerns a parent, is it not then more a problem of the parent, than deviance in the child? Some children are dry at night earlier than others. What is important is that some parents can accept late toilet training better than others. For those who are worried and anxious about a child who still is enuretic at any age, there is not only need to try to understand the particular child, but his parent as well. As we will discuss later, in this instance the parent is the patient rather than the child, although the child is the reason for help being sought.

In attempting to determine if a trait is *normal or abnormal* one must view it in terms of the child's development and in the general cultural and subcultural setting in which it occurs. This includes the culture of the family and the personalities of the parents with their particular qualities, especially their attitudes and personal standards. *In summary, normality is relative.*

In evaluating the normality of a trait, one must ask how it specifically fits into this child's developmental phase. One must note whether it is adequate and appropriate for that time in his development, where it appears in his developmental progress as we compare him against himself and his past, and how the behavior compares to that of peers reared in families where the pattern of life and standards are similar to those of his family.

Another way of evaluating a trait is in terms of the child's attempt to master a situation, to overcome a crisis, to develop autonomy. Is he successful in this, or is it evidence of breakdown and failure to master? Does it represent progress for that child, even though it is viewed as a problem by a parent or teacher; or is it regression, and justly a concern of persons who feel responsible for his well-being and development?

Although it is no longer therapeutically valid to counsel parents that a child will "outgrow" his symptoms, there is truth to the statement that every growing infant and child has some behavior characteristics which appear abnormal and are worrisome, but which are only temporary states, a kind of "normal deviancy." In this sense they are "outgrown" in time.

Normality Tests for Older Children

Anna Freud has suggested several items of behavior which constitute "tests of normality," "tests of a well-functioning ego, and of ego intactness," of the personality for children of school age and upwards, and adults. The tests are helpful in diagnosing mental illness, but not in assessing single traits which may appear deviant, but within the context of a particular child's life are appropriate for him at that time.

Ego functions are appropriate in these age groups when there is evidence that there is progressive development toward the following:

(1) Reality testing is intact. (A person who has an intact ego can distinguish clearly between what is real and what is imagined.) Events and objects are perceived as they are, without distortion by fear or fantasy. Judgment and intelligence are used appropriately; fantasy is used in play but only occasionally as a psychologic mechanism to deal with reality.

(2) Memory is reliable and useful.

(3) The individual knows himself as a person, has accumulated knowledge about himself, and has a feeling of worth.

(4) There is ability to transform the instinctual drives and to integrate and synthesize their deviations with the functions of the ego; to adapt, to control one's impulses, to get along in the world with appropriate and conscious self-control as opposed to inappropriate, automatic and impulsive repetitive actions.

(5) Blind danger and pain is avoided.

(6) Speech is used mainly for communication which is comprehensible to others and which serves the adaptive aims of the ego.

(7) There is logical thought and critical intelligence.

(8) There is an adaptive response to the superego, to one's conscience, but there is not over-obedience in an obsessional and neurotic sense, nor a lack of responsiveness.

(9) A good sense of reality implies that a person knows what his body boundaries are, without a self-conscious attitude about his "self." He is at ease, knows what is his "self" without consciously needing to check up to see who and what he is as a body and a personality. (Drugs, fatigue, anxiety, illness may make a person feel unreal, unself-like. This is why medications to change or influence the mood of children must be used cautiously lest they lead to states of delusion, of depersonalization which frighten the child, particularly an adolescent who is already overly concerned about his body, his health and his development.)

It has been suggested earlier that steps and sequences in the child's development follow recognizable patterns, and that if the pediatrician understands their range of normal variation, and the variety of differences in endowment and in environmental influence, he will be in a better position to assess behavior difficulties. Practically we have found that viewing each child in terms of *his* developmental pattern, through *his* normal vicissitudes and over the course of *his* growing years, helps one to guide parents with some of the perplexing problems they face in child rearing.

For example, a mother who is upset by the increasing demands of her child and who is often in conflict with him about his drive for independence, will be able to feel better if she is helped to understand the reasons for the changing character of the child's relationship. She needs to know that in the earliest period satisfaction of his needs by the parent was the predominant feature of the relationship, and that in succeeding phases of increased independence the child needs help in developing autonomy. A study of a child's progress in development from extreme dependence to independence provides insight for explaining some of his behavior. It also throws light on a mother's need gradually to replace the gratification she derived from serving the dependent child, with gratification to be obtained from watching him achieve independence.

Earlier it was stated that a child progresses from one stage or epoch to another, each representing a particular plateau or normative crisis. Crisis is used here not as something ominous or deviant, but as an expected landmark of significance from which a child may proceed; hopefully forward, but occasionally backward, and frequently standing still for a while, as if to take stock of where he is. The very nature of the difference in each child's coping with developmental crisis signifies individual variability. Some children, like their parents, adapt easily; life seems uneventful. Other children, like their parents, take life hard. They are anxiety prone. The anxiety of parents may be felt by their children and taken up as if by contagion. (The characteristics and meaning of anxiety are discussed later. See pages 133–137.)

In considering the child's development from dependency to emotional self-reliance, from infantilism to body independence, or from egocentricity to companionship, one must bear in mind that one is really analyzing the sequence of development from the id-dominated period of life to those periods which are increasingly more ego and superego controlled.

Viewing various behavioral characteristics developmentally along this schema, one may construct a life chart tracing a particular child's early behavior, from sucking to the time when it becomes adult-planned rational eating; from externally enforced cleanliness to the point when he has self-control over bladder and bowel. One may delineate his behavior from the earliest days of marked dependence on his mother to his later independence in adolescence, connecting his early egocentric views of the world to those of mutuality and companionship with peers; when there is pleasure from work as well as from toys and from playing; and finally, following his sex development from the time when erotic body play constituted a major satisfaction and release to that later period when sexual gratification is derived mainly from relationship to another person as well as from his own body manipulation.

Developmental Profiles

In the sections which follow, we will discuss the nature of the infant and child as he appears normally at various epochs in his development. Coinciding with this we will describe the characteristics of the average or normal parent, especially the mother. Our aim is to show what these people are like, how they interact, how they move ahead developmentally and how on occasion they get emotionally disturbed or even mentally sick. We are concerned with the processes of development both normal and abnormal.

There is an enormous gap between understanding a phenomenon on a theoretical level and being able to use that understanding in a way to make relevant intervention possible. Since it is in the clinical setting that a pediatrician makes use of theory and other guidelines for understanding the dynamics of a particular case and determining the appropriate intervention, we will focus particularly on clinical material as anecdotal illustrations.

The translation of the clinician's conceptual understanding of a situation and the kinds of different behaviors which are brought for his appraisal by parents and others, will be viewed as matters to be considered over time. This is occasioned by the fact that not only does behavior evolve, but psychotherapeutic assistance usually does not result from a one-shot visit or a single suggestion by the physician.

It is unfortunately true that psychotherapeutic intervention, preceded by diagnosis, takes time because both clinician and patient must have opportunity to explore the situation to their mutual satisfaction. As the cases which are described illustrate, the question of timing is of primary importance not only for primary prevention, but even for optimum results therapeutically in what might be called secondary and tertiary prevention. The physician must decide when and under what conditions a patient is ready for a particular kind of assistance and he must know the proper timing, lest the experience be damaging instead of constructive.

Schema of Developmental Charts

To facilitate an understanding of each period of maturation a schema of developmental charts will be shown. These charts approximate the dynamic and viable developments from birth through adolescence which may be expected simultaneously from the child and his parents. From the first moment of extra-uterine life the human organism faces and adapts to the tasks of living in the outside world. Each particular period of maturation encompasses its own special tasks and is associated with certain behavioral characteristics that enhance the accomplishment of those tasks.

Under normal circumstances the process leads to a higher plateau and more complex development. If, however, the expected normal patterns are disrupted or inoperative, development becomes aberrant, with consequent physiologic and/or psychologic conditions of pathology.

The charts delineate the parallel development processes of child and parent in each phase of development; as it proceeds on a normal course, or aberrantly towards minimal or extreme illness.

Normal behavior reaction patterns may never become pathologic. When circumstances decree that a pathologic condition develops, normal patterns may proceed directly to a minimal or to a maximal pathologic condition, or be fixed at some point in between. Reversibility is possible, often without intervention, especially from a minimal pathologic condition back to normal. Many stress reactions are transient and partial regressions to earlier modes of behavior and represent healthy steps in development. However, if the regressions become chronic and more total, they are preludes to severe disease.

The aim of the pediatrician is to prevent a pathologic condition. When this is impossible, his efforts should be directed at facilitating rehabilitation through reversing a pathologic situation. Psychologic development consists of a series of processes which frequently are alterable.

Chapter 2

PREGNANCY

Anticipatory Guidance

A woman usually begins to serve as a mother only after she has become pregnant (only true, of course, in those cases where the child under discussion is the biologic offspring of the mother who faces the problems of child rearing). We therefore begin with pregnancy as the first period in the life of mother and child when the services of a pediatrician may be beneficial from the psychologic and helping point of view.

The usual practice of a pediatrician has been to meet the parents expecting a baby at least once or twice before the delivery. Such an arrangement has proved practical and helpful to all parties concerned. For the pediatrician, it permits evaluation of the parents-to-be as persons, and provides some insight into their personalities, fears, anxieties, aspirations and hopes. For the parents, as they start to know the pediatrician, it brings oportunities to ask questions about infant care, physiology of the newborn, the advantages and disadvantages of breast feeding, and other questions which should be answered constructively so as to prevent a later development of fears and anxieties which might lead to problems in infant care.

Such anticipatory guidance is usually provided after the seventh month of pregnancy. Then the mother wants advice regarding child care in what has been called "the nest-building stage" of her pregnancy. She begins to think of her infant as a special person, fulfilling various fantasies she may have about a baby, or about herself as a mother. At this time many women have fears about the outcome of their pregnancy, the most severe being that the infant will be malformed or stillborn.

Where parents have planned a pregnancy, and have good and adequate medical supervision during the pregnancy period, they usually have feelings of hope and joy, tinged with minor concerns about their ability to provide adequate care for baby. Frequently where the pregnancy has not been planned, and comes at a particularly difficult time

13

in the life of the parents, displeasure may be expressed along with deeper feelings of anger and overt rejection. Since these latter feelings may become the ingredients of a depression antepartum or postpartum, the pediatrician should be on the alert for signs of their appearance.

In the first meeting with parents and in taking the history, it would be helpful to the pediatrician in planning his role to ask some questions about the desirability of the pregnancy, feelings aroused when the pregnancy first became known to the parents, and whether they were enjoying the pregnancy period. Questions about the mother's ability to sleep, the content of any nightmares, her appetite and interest in food, concern about her personal health all may provide some insight into these matters. Questions about the mother's feelings, especially worries, may elicit information about topics such as fear that the baby might be injured in birth, might not be born alive, and the influence of the delivery on her body. Asking a mother whether she plans to nurse the baby, and what motives are involved in her decision will provide the pediatrician with hints as to the type of feeding he should recommend, or to what degree he may anticipate problems around feeding techniques.

Early Signs of Pathology

The psychopathologic condition most dreaded by physicians is a postpartum depression. Mild anxiety is encountered during many pregnancies. This is readily overcome by reassurance or resolution of the precipitating problem. Apprehension about the costs of obstetric and pediatric care, the ability to pay for the extra expense of having a new member of the family, or illness in another member, may appear as precipitating agents. Similarly, a mild form of depression is common 3 or 4 days after delivery, and invariably on the day the mother leaves the hospital to return home with her infant. Usually this is also evanescent. If they are aware of such contingencies, mothers and pediatricians may limit these episodes. The healthy mother readjusts to life at home, particularly if provided with assistance that permits her some days of gradual return to the full-time occupation of running a family.

Some women become excessively concerned for themselves or their families during their pregnancy and some seriously depressed after the birth of the baby. The latter may be characterized as a puerperal depression. From studies of such severely disturbed women, there is evidence to show that often the periods of depression may be anticipated and predicted with accuracy. For example, history of a previous mental disorder, abnormal family or marital relations, an abnormal obstetric or medical history, all suggest particular stress. If the expected date of confinement marks the anniversary of a particularly unhappy period in the life of the mother, it should warn the pediatrician and obstetrician.

In one of our cases, a young woman attempted suicide on the anniversary of her mother's death by self-destruction. Women who have experienced difficulty in a previous pregnancy such as difficult delivery or a stillbirth, or where there has been an acute or severe shortage of money, must be viewed as being predisposed to a depression.

It has been our experience that the pediatrician, and especially the obstetrician, frequently fail to "get the message" from what some of their pregnant women say to them. As a consequence, abnormal conditions are undetected until a catastrophe develops.

The following case is illustrative:

Mrs. R.H., aged 40 years, delivered her second baby prematurely. Six weeks later on days when she came in to minister to the newborn and to make preparations for taking it home, the nurses observed that she seemed confused and lacked the skills expected of a woman who had experience in infant care. On the day we interviewed her, this woman had her 6 weeks postpartum examination and was diagnosed "physically and mentally normal" by her obstetrician. In talking about the new baby to the pediatrician who had been telling her about child care but who had not previously heard any responses from her, Mrs. R.H. seemed confused, slow to react, and when asked about her hearing acuity, she said that she was somewhat deaf. Her lack of ability to understand some simple questions gave the impression that she was emotionally disturbed, probably depressed.

When asked about her physical health, she said that she had been nauseated for quite some time. Asked if this resembled the kind of nausea she had felt in the early weeks of pregnancy, she replied that not only was the symptom the same, but the reason for its existence was identical to that of the previous time. Questioned further, this woman said that she was still pregnant with the second baby and that this was causing her nausea. She said that she had never been asked about her feelings, and that there had never been occasion for her to confide this information to her obstetrician or to the pediatrician. Since this was a fantasy which could not be dispelled by our simply telling her that she was not pregnant, she was referred back to her obstetrician for another pelvic examination. She seemed reassured by his verdict that no fetus remained in the womb.

Suspecting that fantasy was an expression of deep psychopathologic condition, the newborn was kept in the hospital for a longer period of time permitting an arrangement whereby the mother could visit the infant daily, participate in her care, and have conferences with the pediatrician. A friendly relationship was established with the pediatrician which permitted her to talk at length about her life, the pregnancies out of wedlock, her concern about money, her wish to be married, and especially her suspicion that the physicians were interested in removing her firstborn, an idiot, from her care. She said that she had not talked much about herself before, because she wanted to keep her mentally defective child with her and that she would resist all attempts to institutionalize him. When informed that there was no intention to remove her firstborn from her, but rather to help her rear the second and to restore her own health, she became cooperative.

The role of the pediatrician for most women in the last weeks of pregnancy is that of advising them about infant care, the purchase of articles such as clothing, bathinette and diapers. It is not to be expected that a single session devoted to details on these subjects is enough to learn about or to remove feelings of inadequacy. The same subjects should be discussed later, particularly after the birth of the baby when the mother is pressed by her concern to ask specific questions. Guidance then will be especially meaningful.

Probably the most important function of the pediatrician antenatally is to establish a trusting relationship with the mother; to show that he is friendly and accepting of her despite the fears, anxieties and even ambivalence she may demonstrate towards her baby and her husband. Discussion of the fee, the frequency of visits to the physician's office and other matters of business may relieve the parents of some of their concerns about their ability to pay.

If the pediatrician feels that he does not have the time to see such patients individually, groups of women, occasionally accompanied by their husbands, may be dealt with after hours. Such group discussion not only provides the pediatrician an opportunity to answer questions and to give advice, but there often is an exchange of feelings and information which is mutually supportive as well as instructive to the participants. Too frequently it is taken for granted that these women and their husbands understand the anatomy and physiology of their own bodies. Invariably questions of health, body care and sexual intercourse are brought out. The physical nature of the baby seems an item of less worry to them than that of their own physical conditions. Anything which may be done to help women obtain gratification from their pregnancy and infant care will minimize the frequency of their unfounded concern and the development of behavior problems. This is not to say that the infant is to be neglected and his needs go unrecognized. But in the pregnancy period, these needs seem subordinate to those of the mother.

Chapter 3

THE NEWBORN AND YOUNG INFANT
(Birth to 6 months)

THE NEWBORN AND YOUNG INFANT

Tasks in Process

INFANT

To adjust physiologically to extra-uterine life.

To develop appropriate psychologic response.

To assimilate experientially, with increasing capacity to postpone and accept substitutes.

MOTHER

To sustain baby and self physically and pleasurably.

To give and get emotional gratification from nurturing baby.

To foster and integrate baby's development.

Acceptable Behavioral Characteristics

INFANT

Copes with mechanics of life (eating, sleeping, etc.)

Body needs urgent.

Reflexes dominate.

Has biologic unity with mother.

Establishes symbiotic relationship to mother.

Sucking behavior prominent.

Cries when distressed.

Responds to mouth, skin, sense modalities.

Is unstable physiologically.

Functions egocentrically.

Is completely dependent.

Has low patience tolerance.

Is non-cognitive; expresses needs instinctually.

Develops trust in ministering adult.

Begins to "expect."

MOTHER

Provides favorable feeding and handling. Gets to "know" baby.

Develops good working relationship with baby.

Has tolerance for baby.

Promotes sense of trust.

Learns baby's cues.

Applies learning to management of baby.

Interacts emotionally with baby.

Encourages baby's development.

Has reasonable expectations of baby.

18

(Birth to 6 months)

Minimal Psychopathology

INFANT

Feeding and digestive problems.
Sleep disturbances.
Excessive sucking activity.
Excessive motor discharge.
Excessive crying.
Excessive irritability.
Hypertonicity.
Difficult to comfort.

MOTHER

Indifference to baby.
Ambivalence towards baby and its needs.
Self-doubt and anxiety.
Intolerance of baby's characteristics.
Over- or under-responds to baby.
Premature or inappropriate expectations.
Dissatisfaction with role of motherhood.

Extreme Psychopathology

INFANT

Lethargy (depression).
Marasmus.
Cannot be comforted.
Unresponsive.
Infantile autism.
Developmental arrest.

MOTHER

Alienation from baby.
Severe depression.
Excessive guilt.
Complete inability to function in maternal role.
Overwhelming and incapacitating anxiety.
Denies or tries to control baby's needs.
Severe clashes with baby.
Vents life's dissatisfactions on baby.

3

Assessing Adaptation of the Mother-Baby Couple

Strictly speaking the newborn has no psychologic problems. He may be the cause of concern, but the parents, particularly the mother, are the persons in need of help. The newly delivered woman is worried about the physical intactness of her baby and the condition of his health. She is interested in his sex. The pediatrician may be reassuring when he examines the newborn on the bed of the mother, explaining conditions as he goes along, answering her questions, and letting her see for herself the infant's state of health and physical development. Her ambivalent expression, or her negative one, on the sex of the baby should be noted by the pediatrician for it may play some part in her ability to accept the child's sexual role later on.

Rooming-in of baby with mother in the hospital offers opportunities for the couple to know each other. The mother examines her baby, and learns about his patterns of reacting to hunger, satiety, pain, and pleasure. He "gets the feel" of his handler.

Since the general well-being of both baby and mother, as well as the health of both, is dependent on how soon they develop mutual success in the feeding endeavor, the mother should be told in some detail the techniques of feeding whether or not she is a primipara. Such explanations will need to be repeated frequently, more to some women than to others, depending on their health, mood, and experience.

The woman who breast-feeds should anticipate some trouble initially in making contact between baby and nipple, and in the sensation caused by the baby's sucking, which may be a mixture of discomfort and pleasure. If the mother understands that nursing the baby should gratify her, giving her feelings akin to an orgasm, she will be better able to deal with them and without guilt. Permitting the baby to root, to use his hands in feeling the breast and later the face of the mother, should be acceptable and pleasing to the mother. To the baby it provides kinesthetic stimulation, and probably a feeling of affectionate closeness.

The irregularity of the baby's appetite in the first days may alarm some mothers and make them feel that all scheduling of feeding and other child care practices are bound to fail. If the mother can be patient and gradually learn how to coordinate the baby's schedule with one more comfortable to herself and to provide cues for feeding time, she will become more adaptable. Similarly, if a mother is willing to be permissive in giving the infant the amount of food that it needs, and in appropriate form, she will keep him satisfied. Sooner or later he will designate the kind of baby he is in terms of his rhythm of eating and sleeping, and problems will be prevented if the mother can arrange her time in child care to coincide with his rhythm.

Observing the infant's needs in a permissive fashion is not to be considered as spoiling, although some parents will raise the question. If they can be informed about the child's ability to develop greater patience as he grows a little older, mothers will be more accepting of the uncoercive approach in the first weeks of life. They should be helped to understand that later there will be many more appropriate times for teaching him self-discipline by limiting his activities. As we point out subsequently, mothers should be aware of a baby's inborn pattern of reacting to new experiences and to her own way of dealing with such situations. Some babies permit earlier and more strict scheduling than others. Similarly mothers differ in their ability to schedule and to be permissive.

The variety of caretaking procedures in infancy provide many opportunities for the mother to help the child psychologically. Not only as she feeds him appropriately, but as she in addition provides fondling, talks to him, and prevents or reduces pain does she promote his physical health, helps him to learn, and fosters the sense of trust. Removing tension as one feeds a baby who is hungry, providing gentle skin care, helping him to fall asleep readily, promote a satisfactory relationship between mother and baby. These things as a rule provide gratification to the mother as well as to the infant.

Where a good working relationship fails to be accomplished, the babies are irritable, present problems of eating and retaining food, cry excessively, and often are termed *hypertonic*. The term itself characterizes behavior such as excessive crying, crying without apparent provocation, difficulty in falling asleep, restless sleep, an exaggerated startle reaction. Hypertonicity unquestionably in some instances is due to the baby's biologic make-up. But having said that, we know little about what is meant by significance of the behavior. Nevertheless it is true that some babies from birth and for the first several months of life are jittery, sleep lightly, have trouble releasing into sleep, regurgitate and have diarrhea. Not only does this behavior worry a mother, because she may think of the infant as being sick, but it raises doubts in her mind about her own ability to care for him successfully. Such doubt, guilt and worry may make it difficult for her to handle the baby with ease and with pleasure. Her attitude compounds the baby's difficulties. Such parents often lose sleep for many days, and the baby fails to thrive.

At this point a pediatrician can be most helpful in examining the baby, determining its state of health, prescribing whatever remedies seem indicated, and reassuring the mother verbally. Bringing in parent substitutes to help in some of the baby care may relieve the mother, especially if she can rest during the time of separation. However, some mothers take such suggestions as an implication that the pediatrician has found fault with them and is suggesting a permanent substitute.

The pediatrician who tells a mother that these are not his evaluations, but that he is motivated by sympathy for her, usually can change her guilt into a more rational attitude.

As the child's appetite is satisfied, he is able to tolerate periods of hunger longer and to take in greater amounts of food which tide him over for longer periods of time. In this way he lengthens his own feeding interval, and schedules himself to a three meal a day pattern. Along with this, his sleeping pattern becomes more scheduled and regular. Sometimes after the third or fourth month of such sleeping regularity, many infants develop wakefulness late in the evening, after initially falling asleep. They awake abruptly, usually do not seem hungry, cry until handled and eventually fall asleep. There may be another or several reawakenings during the night. Covering them or changing the diaper may be enough to reassure them, but a parent, who does not understand the usualness of this sleep pattern, may in anxiety overdo the holding and cuddling, overstimulate, and perpetuate the sleep problem beyond its usual course.

The infant several months old will already have learned the comfort obtained from sucking fingers or fist. This should not be denied him. Where a mother for one reason or another cannot accept this habit and tries forcibly to end it, she may actually intensify it. There may be a spillover into other behavioral traits which are annoying to her, such as excessive crying, difficulty of falling asleep and continued wakefulness. Such mothers also are intolerant of rubber pacifiers, although others who are more relaxed are willing for babies to use them to overcome discomfort or to induce sleepiness.

A less frequent complaint than when the baby is overactive is that he is lethargic. Many mothers enjoy a baby that is "good," meaning that he makes few demands on them and spends much time in sleep. This may be normal. There are infants with placid dispositions already manifest at birth. On the other hand, it may be a pathologic condition and if it is, mothers should not be told something to the contrary. Particularly unfortunate is the prediction to parents that a baby "will outgrow" a trait, when there's no evidence to substantiate the prediction, or worse when there is evidence of a pathologic condition which will be long-lasting.

Assessing Signs of Pathology

The perceptive pediatrician need not be at a loss to recognize abnormality in an infant. There are usually clear clinical signs as well as several simple developmental procedures which may provide clues. For example, noting position of the head whether it sags or is held steady; what are the position of the hands? Are they used in grasping, raking and for prehension as one would expect? Does the baby coo, laugh, smile, and listen to his own vocalization? Or does he lie impassively and without interest when spoken to? The eyes should be examined to find out whether they regard the observer's face, whether they are used in observing hands or toys, or in expressing expectation in feeding situations. The eyes tell much about the attentiveness or inattentiveness (lethargy).

The lethargic infant warrants a thorough developmental examination, preferably by specialists. Even the pediatrician may get important clues from examining the baby following the schema for infant observation and developmental examination (see Chapter 8).

A baby may be lethargic because he is understimulated. In taking a history, one finds that some mothers are afraid to handle their babies and leave them to themselves for long periods of time except when feeding or changing them. Others find it difficult to talk to their babies, because they seem "unintelligent and not like an adult." The baby who prattles and coos pleases most mothers, assures her that he is healthy and developing normally. Occasionally a woman cannot take this amount of "noise." One of our patients recently bought earstoppers so that she could be spared both the prattle of her baby and the need to reply. This information not only tells much about the personality of the mother, but is predictive of certain problems which may come from a faulty baby-mother relationship.

One of the most serious of these is a condition known as *infantile autism* (see page 209). While there probably are many causes for this psychopathologic state, in a fair number of cases it is associated with underhandling by mothers who are depressed by their child's unresponsiveness or in other ways are incapable of giving of their personal and emotional selves to their infants. A baby whose talk is recognized by the mother and who responds with speech not only gives him pleasure, but fosters language development in him.

Infants who are born with certain physical deficiencies, such as blindness, deafness, or kinesthetic impairment of skin surface because of extensive skin disease, need to obtain other sensory gratification to make up the deficits. Encouraging a blind baby to use his fingers in self-feeding, to feel the face of his mother, as well as other objects like toys, not only teaches him something, but gives him sensory pleasure which is important for his physical, intellectual, social and emotional development. Babies with extensive lesions of the skin require more cuddling, more opportunities to use their eyes and ears in order to make up for the lack of kinesthetic stimulation, or to counteract the unpleasantness of excessive itching and pain which may come from their skin disturbance. Some babies require more time at feeding, as well as more sucking, since they are denied sensory stimulation from other modalities.

Similarly, infants restricted physically by casts or splints should be provided with satisfactions coming from contact with people, as well as with sights and sounds, to help overcome the ill effects of immobilization.

The mutual give and take between mother and child can be furthered or discouraged when supplementary feedings have started. A baby's efforts to feed himself are encouraged as the mother accepts his blundering efforts as an essential part of the feeding process. This fosters independence.

However, if self-feeding is urged or coerced prematurely, especially if it is done for the purpose of making him clean or fostering an independence of which he is not yet capable, the baby will be discouraged with his failure to please. He may become negative and obstinate. The feeding problems which are more or less normal for all children as they learn new skills in feeding, may be more severe when complicated by a clash of wills. As the mother's anger mounts, the baby may get the feeling of not being loved any longer. He may be puzzled by the change in attitude of the parent and show his disturbance in other ways such as in crying excessively, not eating, or in disturbed sleep. In such a somatic response to psychologic stress, the physician should be cautious in labeling the condition "psychosomatic," lest the mother be made anxious by the implication that a psychopathologic condition of a deep and lasting variety is in the making. Such a psychopathologic situation as a rule does not arise from a single experience.

In essence then, "behavior problems" in the newborn period are primarily psychologic problems *in the mother* who misinterprets the normal physical condition of her infant, or attempts to speed up his development and force him to do things before he is ready. The infant needs to have his instinctual demands satisfied. From this comes gratification to the mother as well because she has served her baby satisfactorily. When her own personality interferes with meeting the infant's demands, or does not permit her to be gratified by her own successful ministrations, one must then assess her personality for clues to the origin of the problems. A woman may be attempting to rear her child without the help of a husband; she may be depressed; she may be preoccupied with concerns of making a living or adjusting to her own health; she may be lonely and attempt to overinterpret or oversatisfy the child's demands. This leads to an unusual closeness and breeds a demanding attitude in the infant even at this early period in his life. Such mothers may complain of problems but be non-accepting of help because their unconscious mechanisms militate against accepting help.

The Premature Infant

Any form of defect in a newborn baby is a severe shock to his parents. Prematurity is no exception. Even when the child has a good chance of survival and normality, the mother is almost sure to feel that she has failed to do this important thing well and that she has disappointed her husband. In addition, she wonders whether she will be able to take proper care of this fragile being whom she has neither held nor nourished and who seems to belong entirely to others, segregated in a special nursery.

Even under the most favorable circumstances most women suffer some degree of postpartum depression. This feeling of let-down is almost invariably intensified after a premature birth. Not only is the mother disappointed and anxious, she is distressed because she may not have felt the surge of maternal warmth for her child which she had expected. Without a chance to hold him and gain intimate knowledge of her child, unable to feel pride in what she has brought forth, she is handicapped from the start.

The longer she must wait to make the baby her own, the heavier the sense of estrangement becomes. The hardest moment of all is when she leaves the hospital and unlike the other mothers has nothing to take home with her.

Nowadays women do not take their motherliness for granted and have become self-conscious about it. Neither is the quality of motherliness manifest in one easily recognizable form. It varies at different periods of their own and their children's growth. Some women who intensely enjoy a baby are miserable with a 4 year old. Others who genuinely love the company of small children and know instinctively how to win them are frustrated and angry at the vagaries of their adolescents. Nobody has told the mother who is beset by self-doubt, that her neighbor who seems to love all her children all of the time probably also suffers moments of despair and failure as a parent.

The best way a doctor can help the mother of a premature baby is to give her generous doses of emotional support. Instead of crude attempts at cheeriness while on the run to his next appointment, he will do her a great service if he can encourage her to talk of her sense of failure and depression. Only when he has listened will he be in a position to assure her that these feelings are natural and will pass, though it may take a while. When her baby goes home and she learns, as she will to care for him, she will get much satisfaction from his growth and change. Then she will find that she is as good a mother as any.

If the chances for a premature infant's survival seem poor, the doctor must reveal his doubts to the parents, lest if the baby dies, they suffer another blow, and in addition a sense of betrayal by the doctor who they felt had encouraged them to believe their child would live. At the same time, the measures being taken to save the child should be described to them so that they know that everything possible is being done—and that the doctor truly cares.

Mrs. S., who was 7½ months pregnant, gave birth to a male baby weighing 4 pounds. Sixteen months earlier she had given birth to a 5 month nonviable infant, also male, who died immediately. Naturally enough, this second premature birth plunged Mrs. S. into grief and depression—especially because this time, after she had passed the seventh month, her hopes were high for carrying the child to term. Now she was convinced that he too would die and that she was destined never to fulfill her dream of a "real family." Her husband, she told the doctor, wanted children almost more than she did.

Since there is some familial tendency toward miscarriage and prematurity the doctor felt unable to give Mrs. S. complete reassurance that her chances for more live births were as good as the average. She raised the question of subsequent children almost at once. "I suppose it's always going to be this way," she had said. "I just cannot ever bring a healthy child into the world and shouldn't even try." The doctor replied that this was not necessarily true, that she might indeed have normal full-term babies and that more about the causes and prevention of prematurity is being discovered. He reminded her that this time she had had a live child whose chances seemed good. He was optimistic, but it was still too early to be certain.

Mrs. S. still cried a good deal, seemed uninterested when she saw the infant through the nursery window and on the day she went home responded listlessly when her husband suggested they go say a temporary good-bye to their baby. Both of them visited the child in the 3 weeks that followed and Mrs. S. began to relax a bit when it seemed more and more sure that he would live. Mr. S. had always been optimistic but he was also sympathetic to his wife's misgivings and considerate of her state of mind.

When after a month the baby weighed almost 5 pounds, and was getting along, he was discharged. The mother had visited the nursery daily to become accustomed to giving him his care and when she took him home Mrs. S. seemed more confident and happy than she had been. Yet she soon presented a problem for the pediatrician. No matter how often he assured her that the baby was doing well and that it took many months for a premature child to catch up with others their age, Mrs. S. fussed and worried. Telephone calls were constant. Even when the child achieved 10 pounds and was obviously healthy and lively she devoted her whole time to him. Her social life with her husband and all out-of-home activities seemed at a standstill.

After 5 months of this, the pediatrician intervened. He asked both Mr. and Mrs. S. to the office at the time when the baby was due for a check-up visit. He expressed his delight at the child's health and growth and called attention to the normality of reflexes, muscle tone and general responsiveness. He then asked the parents how they were feeling after what must have been a long haul. Mr. S. then took over, replying that they were both tired and in need of a change. He would like to take his wife away on a vacation, but she did not feel that she could leave the baby. The doctor then turned to Mrs. S., tactfully inviting her to say how she felt. She had little to say and seemed a bit defensive. The doctor and Mr. S. thereupon discussed various details of where they might go, who could be left in charge of the baby, and what friends were nearby who might drop in to see that all was well. The visit ended with no definite advice given and nothing settled. However Mrs. S. looked happy when she left, as though she realized that even a good mother and even the mother of a premature baby can, with some planning, occasionally leave and enjoy herself elsewhere.

Mr. and Mrs. S. did go away on a trip. Mrs. S.'s mother stayed with the baby in her absence and all went well. The vacation seemed a turning point, apparently proving to Mrs. S. that her child would not vanish if she looked away for a moment. From then on, phone calls were fewer, she handled her baby with assurance and at the end of a year her joy and pride in her son were unmistakable. The doctor also learned that she had consulted her obstetrician about the advisability of another pregnancy.

Discussion. This woman was fortunate in having both a husband and doctor who were patient, practical and emotionally supportive in seeing her through a hard year. Her depression and insecurity were somewhat more severe than most, but not unusual.

As for another pregnancy the doctor would do well to be frank about his estimate of her chances of a successful outcome. Then the choice must be made by the couple themselves who may or may not want to take a calculated risk. But he must also avoid giving the feeling that his unwillingness to urge them to go ahead means that he is actually discouraging them. He should say in effect "If you do decide to go ahead, we will do everything possible to see you through. If you decide not to, that's all right too. You are no less of a woman if you only have one child—and it doesn't have to be a disaster for the child either.

A doctor learns in the course of practice that not every woman who says she wants another baby really is eager to rear an actual flesh and blood child with all the adjustments this involves. Sometimes she is merely trying to prove something about her own ability to carry a pregnancy through; or to bind her husband more closely; or to demonstrate something to her parents or her in-laws. She is unlikely to admit or even be conscious of her hidden motives which are likely to be obscure and complicated. But in time she may herself make the discovery that after all her family is quite satisfactory as it is, and that life offers opportunities and satisfactions other than child-bearing. The urge for yet another pregnancy may then evaporate, and she can take what she already has in peace, and go forward to a life suited to her own needs.

Assignment of Gender in Anatomic Sex Ambiguity (Hermaphroditism)

Regardless of genetic, gonadal and somatic sex, the way a person is reared in the first few years of life largely determines his sexual self-identity. That is to say, psychosexual development and gender role are much more influenced by how a child is dressed, what toys he is given to play with, and of what sex he is regarded by parents and others.

In those individuals with anatomic defects whose rearing emphasizes one gender while the anatomic state gives a sense of another, there is inevitable confusion and eventual psychologic trauma. For this reason it is important that every infant be assigned a sex, preferably within the neonatal period. Where the ambiguity of sex is such that surgical and other examinations are needed to clarify the anatomic and physiologic status, these procedures should be performed within the first few months, if possible, so that a sex may be assigned and never thereafter altered. Since the physician is best equipped to judge the physiologic considerations, he has the responsibility of sex determination. He must then thoroughly discuss the sex assignment and his reasons for it with the parents. Their concurrence is essential in order to provide the optimal development and ultimate function consistent with the assigned sex of rearing.

In making sex assignments of infant hermaphrodites, an assignment should be avoided for which surgical repair of the genitalia is impossible. For example, male pseudo-hermaphrodites who have a phallus which will not be functional should not be reared as males but as females. Infrequently male pseudo-hermaphrodites have a phallus which will be functional and they should be reared as males, with surgical removal of the uterus and tubes, and repair of the hypospadias, chordee, and scrotal cleft. All female pseudo-hermaphrodites should be reared as females.

When the diagnosis of hermaphroditism is made after early infancy, the question of a change in the sex or rearing often arises. While rearing may be changed before the age of 2 years without causing confusion of gender role, after that age it is best to continue to rear the child in keeping with the originally assigned sex. Psychosexual differentiation usually has advanced to the point of no return by the time a child is ready for school. By adolescence, the child who has been reared to consider himself one sex gender and to assume that role, usually finds it impossible to adjust to a new role which has been assigned him anatomically by surgery. He will continue to behave sexually as he has been taught to behave from the earliest years. This may label him a homosexual and subject him to the unhappiness and hazards that go with such labeling. He may even demand further surgical change to make him more anatomically compatible with his assigned gender.

In determining the proper sex assignment among older children, especially adolescents, extensive interviews with the child alone, and with his parents, are required so that the child may have assistance in expressing his preferences for the kind of person he wishes to be sexually.

Chapter 4

THE OLDER INFANT
(6 to 18 months)

THE OLDER INFANT

Tasks in Process

INFANT

To develop more reliance and self control.

To differentiate self from mother.

To make developmental progress.

MOTHER

To provide a healthy emotional and physical climate.

To foster weaning, training, habits.

To understand, appreciate and accept baby.

Acceptable Behavioral Characteristics

INFANT

More stable physiologically.

Heightened voluntary motor activity and exploration.

Higher level of patience tolerance.

Instinctual needs in better control.

Strong selective tie to mother.

Stranger differentiation.

Increased verbality, play and sensori-motor behavior.

Discernible social responses; joyful in play.

Outbursts of negativism and anger.

Sensory modalities important.

Emergence of idiosyncratic patterns.

Demonstrates memory and anticipation.

Begins to imitate.

MOTHER

Derives satisfaction from serving baby well.

Responds appropriately to baby's signs of distress.

Aware of baby's inborn reaction pattern.

Has more confidence in own ability.

Gives positive psychologic reassurance (fondling, talking, comforting).

Shows pleasure in baby.

Keeps pace with baby's advances.

Is accepting of baby's idiosyncracies.

(6 to 18 months)

Minimal Psychopathology

INFANT

Excessive crying, anger and irritability.
Low frustration tolerance.
Excessive negativism.
Finicky eater, sleep disturbances.
Digestive and elimination problems.
Noticeable motility patterns (fingering, rocking, etc.).
Delayed development.

MOTHER

Disappointed in and unaccepting of baby.
Misses baby's cues.
Infancy unappealing.
Impersonal management.
Attempts to coerce to desired behavior.
Over-anxious or over-protective.
Mildly depressed and apathetic.

Extreme Psychopathology

INFANT

Tantrums and convulsive disorders.
Apathy, immobility and withdrawal.
Extreme and obsessive finger-sucking, rocking, head-banging.
No interest in objects, environment or play.
Anorexia.
Megacolon.
Inexpressive of feeling.
No social discrimination.
No tie to mother; wary of all adults.
Infantile autism.
Failure to thrive.
Arrested development.

MOTHER

Neglect or abuse of baby.
Rejection of the maternal role.
Severe hostility reactions.
No attempt to understand or gratify baby.
Deliberately thwarts infant.
Complete withdrawal and separation from baby.

Expected Development and/or Incipient Problems

After several weeks of experience together, mother and baby usually show great skill in adapting to each other. The need for mutuality of interests continues, and so does the need for a mother to still abide by and foster the dependent state of the baby. However, from 6 months onward, the infant takes dramatic developmental steps. He continues to make demands because of his instinctual needs, but he is better able to control them. Most mothers have by now developed confidence in themselves and realize that in meeting the baby's needs, there is no longer the urgency to anticipate them and avoid entirely making him wait. Most mothers enjoy this period of babyhood. Occasionally some find it less appealing because the infant is still "so much of a baby," unlike an adult to whom one can talk or relate.

As the baby enters the second half of the first year of life, his motor development has progressed to a point where he no longer is content to lie on his back for long periods of time. He uses arms and legs to bring pleasure to himself from the simple movements, and also to change his position, cruise about, to crawl and finally to walk. He may flail his limbs about in anger and have crying temper tantrums which are sometimes accompanied by breath-holding spells. These spells are frightening to parents who consider them a convulsive disorder, and even fear that the baby may stop breathing. These periods of unconsciousness are momentary and mothers may be reassured when told that no harm results from them.

Prevention is possible when one tries to find out why a baby must resort to such extreme measures to get what he wants and when one copes more satisfactorily with his needs. Is the mother missing his cues for feeding, for being dry and clean, for being tended-to after a long sleep? Is she too stimulating or demanding in correcting his efforts to feed himself? Does the baby have an unusually short patience tolerance? Already in early infancy a baby shows his aggression by biting and by angry crying. While these are unsettling, and annoying episodes to parents, they represent energy and liveliness. More serious is the opposite state when outbursts of anger occur infrequently or not at all. Such a child may be viewed as being either physically sick or mentally retarded.

Refusal to eat solid foods may stem from unwillingness to bite or swallow either because of pain or a negative attitude on the part of the baby. Negativism may follow too much urging and coaxing to eat properly. The baby continues to get great pleasure from biting, tasting, sucking and chewing, as he did at a younger age. The sense of satisfaction gained in using these mechanisms to express anger is also manifest. Another feeding problem may be anorexia, unwillingness to eat any foods, or drink milk, for hours or days. Psychologically speaking, this also may be a period of holding out or negativism; or it may be apathy in a child who has been neglected. It is as if the child is turning his feelings of aggression and disappointment against himself. The first inclination in anger is to foist it on his mother or on other objects. But where he has been consistently deprived of affection, adequate care, and the opportunity to be satisfied by the ministrations of people, he goes from anger to depression.

Important landmarks developmentally in the period beginning with the last months of the first year and extending into the second year are those of speech development, improved motor coordination, sphincter control, and a change in play patterns. Not only does the complexity of behavior increase with development, but the nature of the psychologic problems change as does their complexity. The role of the mother continues to be paramount in a baby's development or his lack of it. She is the person, along with the husband to some extent, who views with alarm, complains of problems and comes for help.

The infant, as it were, is attempting to deal with his developmental problem through his body. He cries, kicks, bites, vomits, withholds feces and does not sleep. And as he does this, he evokes anxiety, anger, resentment, apprehension and other emotions in the mother. Some of the behavior problems common to the period will be discussed in the succeeding pages.

Normal Separation Anxiety

During the last third of the first year, though it may be a bit earlier or later, an important change in a child's emotional life may be observed. Even those infants who heretofore have readily accepted all comers now become shy and refuse the attentions of anyone but their mothers or familiar persons. This "8-month anxiety" varies in intensity from child to child. Some show it merely by staring critically at a stranger. Others are clearly terrified upon not seeing mother and give way to disconsolate wails, screams, and desperate clinging to the mother on seeing her.

Unless prolonged, this behavior is not abnormal. It marks the point at which the child, though able earlier than this to distinguish his mother's face, now has come definitely to prefer hers above all others and to depend on it exclusively. For the infant's healthy emotional development, the mother's face is of extreme importance. He sees it as ensuring food, warmth, approval, play and relief from discomfort. It means "all's well with the world."

This deep early attachment first to the mother, then to one or two other familiar people who remain fixtures during his early years, is believed by psychologists to provide the basis for all love relationships.

4

Enforced maternal separations of short or long duration such as during illness, often are upsetting and lead to a temporary estrangement from the mother when she returns. Mothers frequently cannot understand this. Assuming that the child missed her and cried at her absence, then why does he not accept her return with pleasure and joy. But the child now feels uncertain of her, needing to prove that she will really stay this time. He cannot bear to invest in an intense relationship with her, lest she once more disappears and he again must face the grief of parting. Of course, an infant and toddler does not consciously think this way. But from many observations of children in psychotherapy, where there has been maternal separation, they have responded as described. It is apparent that even babies *feel* like older children *think*. Older children grieve when bereft of the presence and love of a person to whom they have been particularly close. A child subjected to loss of a person to whom he is particularly close emotionally, or to a series of losses, may be unable to establish close emotional ties to other persons for a long time, if ever. (See Fatal and Incurable Illness pp. 238–239.)

Where a child is suddenly deprived of his mother for a long period of time without someone in his life who holds him, cuddles him, smiles at and plays with him, he may become depressed, stop learning, regress to less mature levels and show other signs of serious disturbance.

Normally, a child outgrows this exclusive demand for his mother by gradually discovering that even when she leaves him she can be counted on to return soon—and that others around him are also friendly and dependable. But irritability or inconsistent handling by the mother— such as desperate angry discipline alternating with equally desperate over-indulgence, increase the child's anxiety and tend to prolong this phase of growth. Often the mother's failure is born of fatigue and "housewife blues." But mostly it results from her not understanding that a certain amount of separation anxiety along with nighttime wakefulness is to be expected and will run a normal course if she takes it easy, accepts some of it, but also watches for opportunities to help the child grow beyond it.

The Case of Christine B.

Presenting Complaint. Christine, aged 10 months (40 weeks), adopted by the family when 3 months old, was hospitalized for 4 days at the advice of a family pediatrician. Admitting cause: sleep disturbance.

Family Background:

      Father, age 40 — electrical engineer

      Mother, age 34 — formerly laboratory technician

      Brother, age 2½ — (also adopted) health no problem

For several weeks Christine has waked at night screaming in great distress and inconsolable. Her mother has gone to her, held and tried many ways of comforting her, but the child has loudly resisted all attempts to be put down or left alone.

The mother further tells us that when Christine first came to her adoptive home, she was pronounced a healthy active infant by the family physician. The mother, however, felt that at first Christine seemed "remote," and "unattached." This characteristic soon changed; she became fiercely attached to her new mother demanding to be constantly held *only* by her mother. In her absence, however, the child found her father a satisfactory, unfrightening substitute.

Though active and agile, Christine plays with only a few toys and without great interest. Though there have been no special problems between her and her brother, if there is a tussle over a toy, Christine is almost always a quick winner.

Toilet training had not yet been attempted though the mother sometimes tried to "catch" her bowel movements in a potty chair, but there was no insistence on this.

Clearly, Christine's mother seemed tense and overwrought—exhausted from lack of sleep plus the feeling that she had mismanaged and was to blame for the child's difficulties. Now she wanted expert advice and help.

Examination and Hospital Findings. At admission, Christine was found essentially healthy. Blood studies, urinalysis, tuberculin skin test, paper chromatography urine test (routine) were negative.

On psychologic tests, Christine's maturational level averaged at the 44- to 46-week level except for language. In the areas of adaptation, language and personal-social development, she ranged from a 32- to a 56-week level. She was uninterested in toys. Speech consisted of a few repetitive sounds. She responded to her name; hearing seemed unimpaired. In fact one had the impression that she was unusually sensitive to the sounds and visual stimuli of the external world and could not find ways to cope with it.

The child smiled readily, eager to go to anyone who approached the crib and "melted into the arms" of a strange physician who examined her. But if left alone, she stood screaming to be taken up and the nurses were instructed to yield to these demands for a while—then taper off their attentions as the child grew more accustomed to her mother's absence and new surroundings.

In the hospital, Christine slept well at night without waking, daytime demands diminished and during the last days of her stay screamed to be held only by her mother when she visited. This is a common and healthy phenomenon showing that the child's attachment to her mother—worth preserving at all costs—is deeply rooted.

Impressions. The child has normal intelligence. At present she suffers from acute separation anxiety in relation to the mother. It seems likely that her anxiety at being separated from her even momentarily and her strenuous rejection of strange people and places came in more intense form than with most children. In Christine's case this in part may well be due to an innate hyperacute perception of sound and visual stimuli in addition to the traumatic effects of adjusting to a new mother when adopted at the age of 3 months. Christine seemed to fear that she might again lose this source of love and so was at first distrustful ("detached") and later fiercely possessive. Though Christine may be said to have an innate predisposition to anxiety, her hypersensitivity could well become a personality asset if, as time goes on, she can learn to handle it.

The "sleep problem," of which this child showed no signs when in the hospital, would seem to be merely a part of the generalized anxiety. Christine had had a cold and some discomfort from teething when the night-time screaming first started and this disturbed her sleep. Once awake in a dark room, she reacted as she always had upon finding herself alone, *i.e.* with anxiety and loud demands for mother.

The mother was seen twice during the child's 4-day hospitalization. She was assured that Christine was essentially normal mentally and physically and that she herself had made no fatal errors. The frequency and normality of "separation anxiety" at this age were explained in detail and time allowed for her to ask questions and digest the information.

The mother was also encouraged to describe her fatigue as the result of her disturbed nights. Gradually, too, she became willing to talk about Christine being an adopted child. When asked if she ever considered returning her to the adoption agency, she admitted that the thought had occurred in moments of great fatigue but that with equilibrium regained, she knew how much she loved the child and could not possibly part with her.

Suggestions were made on how to introduce Christine to a baby sitter. If someone comes to stay with Christine, the mother should plan to stay around for awhile until the child begins to play with her new friend happily and trustfully. Then when the mother departs some crying is not too serious. The mother should never "sneak out," but tell the child casually she is leaving and will be back soon. She might wave from the street while the child watches from the window and perhaps bring a little present when she returns. It was explained that Christine needs gradually to learn to accept other people and relinquish her exclusive dependence— and that she herself should have more freedom to come and go.

It was explained too that a child is often helped to develop trust in a mother's dependability through games of "go-away-and-come-back," such as peek-a-boo. Mother covers her face, the child pulls the cover off again and again. Or she disappears behind a door, the child pulls it back and rediscovers her smiling face.

The father's important relation to the whole situation was also emphasized. If he can find time to do more in the way of day time play with the child, he is likely to become a more acceptable substitute for the mother at night. Then, if they take turns responding to call, the mother could get some nights of unbroken sleep.

At the final interview, the doctor told the mother that it was important for him to see her again in 6 weeks so as to see how things were going. If that was impossible, then he would call her on the phone for a report. This kind of support, interest and continued willingness to help can be a large factor in restoring a mother's self-confidence and pleasure in her child. Now she can feel she has a friend in the doctor who "understands" and will stand by her.

Follow-Up Discussion. Following discharge from the hospital Christine developed a slight diarrhea; her nights were disturbed, but under these circumstances, the mother felt entirely justified in going to her and comforting her. Thereafter, Christine became "a different baby"— far happier and easier to manage. Such improvements in children following an illness have often been noted and are probably due to the mother's willingness to give in a more generous and conflict-free spirit.

Upon recovery, Christine did of course try out again some of her old ways. She waked now and then and demanded "up." But by now her father was acceptable to the child at night and proved to be a rather helpful partner. As predicted, quiet happy play-time with Christine when he came home in the evening and on weekends did much to give him a secure place in Christine's affections. Not only did the mother get more sleep and some recreation in the daytime when a sitter took over, but she felt she had learned to "take the baby better." This seemed to mean that she had less inner conflict and guilty feelings about going to Christine when needed and also about leaving her to others. Previously she was uncertain on both counts and the resulting tension was perhaps more a cause of fatigue and depression than the actual loss of sleep.

Now she is happier about the child and about herself as a mother. The child has reacted to this change by being more at peace; the waking at night is diminishing and she is more quickly satisfied and willing to be left. Sometime she even stops crying when the mother or father simply call from their bedroom to say they are nearby, but are not coming in.

As has been suggested, what may appear in young children as excessive and intolerable demands must always be considered in the light of a particular child's temperament, history and stage of development. Christine is an adopted child—one who has already lost a mother-person (in the foster home of the first 3 months). Such an experience reinforces the fears with which nearly all children are beset—that they may lose their mothers and so be alone and helpless. They therefore cling (psychologically speaking) to the mother and regard strangers as a threat to their security.

In Christine's case, we have an exceptionally sensitive and perceptive child. Further she is around 10 months old, an age at which fear of the loss of the mother and need for constant reassurance is most marked. A mother needs to understand these things so that she will see her child not as merely "spoiled" (as she is likely to have been told), but as a child going through a phase of development which may be inconvenient but is not unhealthy. She needs to know that her child needs gradual weaning from dependence. To this end, she will need patient persistence.

Though Christine and her mother gained much from the hospital experience, it may be questioned whether this step was necessary. The differential diagnosis, psychologic tests, skilled professional observation and parental counseling might all have been done by the pediatrician in his office or in out-patient clinic. The physician must himself be aware, and help the parents understand too, that time thus spent on "non-medical" matters is not time wasted. On the contrary, in this type of case, wise management is the essence of effective therapy. Maternal relaxation cannot be ordered, it must be induced; and it depends on building the mother's self confidence and ease in daily management. To this end, sympathetic rapport between patient and doctor is the foundation on which the whole procedure rests.

Failure to Thrive in Infants

Infants who fail to thrive without a demonstrable physical reason are not infrequently found in an average pediatric practice. They may come from any of the three main social classes. After diagnostic tests have ruled out a physical pathologic condition as the cause (see Modified Schema page 45), efforts should be made to discover possible relationships to personalities of the persons caring for the baby and the techniques used, particularly in such matters as feeding. Parents are momentarily reassured when told that the physician's diagnostic tests are negative for physical disease, but they soon show guilt at the implication that their child-care practices are faulty, or that something psychologic may be responsible.

The most seriously ill infants who fail to thrive are those whose weight is consistently below the third percentile according to the Stuart Growth Charts. They may or may not be small in stature also. There may be a variety of feeding problems especially vomiting, diarrhea, irritability and anorexia. Inasmuch as these babies have been chronically undersized, and have not responded to a variety of feeding changes, thorough study usually demands hospitalization for a period of several days to a few weeks. Not only does this provide an opportunity for assessment of the baby's condition, but for repeated interviewing of the parents and a detailed search for psychologic, etiologic factors.

When in hospital the parents are encouraged to spend considerable time with their baby in order that the staff may witness the manner of their relationship to the baby, and their techniques of his care. Nurses check up on the daily weight, feeding patterns, and general physiologic and psychologic reactions. It may not take long to find that the parents are using faulty techniques of feeding, or feeding impersonally, as by use of a propped bottle or in not giving enough food to meet caloric needs. In our experience many of these babies are not held or talked to at the time of being fed, at diapering, or when put down to sleep.

Failure to thrive may appear at any age from early infancy to the pre-school period. Since physical, especially neurologic and metabolic examinations and x-ray pictures fail to uncover any significant physical abnormalities for the failure to gain weight and to grow, attention is given to interviewing the parents for their family backgrounds, for information about the parent-infant relationships, the relationship between husband and wife, and the previous success or failure in childrearing.

A detailed personal history of the patient is obtained in the usual manner. However, more attention is given than usual to attempting to detect the nature of the feelings and attitudes of the parents towards the baby and towards life in general. Financial insecurity, unemployment, inadequate housing, marital conflicts, illegitimate pregnancies, physical and mental health problems in parents are some of the conditions which contribute to difficulty in nurturing the child. Invariably the mother herself was deprived of good nurturing in her childhood because of a chaotic home situation, death or illness of her mother, mental illness in one or both parents.

On interviewing the mothers of these babies they frequently appear depressed and anxious; the fathers seem minimally involved in the life of their families, because of disinterest, emotional ill health, or occupation which removes them from the home for long periods of time. In the upper middle-class, infant care may be entirely left to a nursemaid, or a series of them, who treats the baby impersonally and deprives him of consistently affectionate supportive care.

Studies of these families show that frequently the baby's mother had an unusual pregnancy and delivery because of ill health or lack of good obstetric care. The anticipated perception that she had of her baby was incorrect. She was disappointed in the pregnancy and in the offspring. As the baby's temperament and personality either displeased her or affected her in other ways, the mother responded to it with rejection, and more or less neglect. Even a normal, vigorous and active baby to some of these mothers seemed hypertonic and "nervous." The mothers characterized themselves as tense, high-strung, and easily angered. Occasionally these babies were described as being too placid, too quiet and undemanding. It is not surprising then that their mothers on examination proved to be quiet, passive and depressed.

As a consequence of the mother's attitude and feelings, handling was kept at a minimum and the baby's growth and development responded in kind. When tested by developmental examinations generalized delay in development with unevenness in all sectors was characteristic. These babies seemed to have trouble in their relationships to people, demonstrating an unusual watchfulness for such young babies, a lack of cuddleness, delayed smiling and inadequate vocalization. They were not appropriately afraid of strangers, and they were indiscriminate in their acceptance of people they did not know. Gross motor development was delayed in most instances.

The prognosis is good in these babies if parents are able to make changes in their management, and are patient. The pediatrician has a great opportunity to provide a service which gives dramatic results. Since many mothers are unable to minister to their babies because they do not understand the baby's needs, or the proper techniques to satisfy them, the physician's role is one of providing information and teaching the mother. If illness or other reasons prevent the mother from participating actively in the care of the child on a full-time basis, a competent substitute should be found.

The babies are to be given not only the food they need, and in proper amounts, but appropriate stimulation by handling, bathing, cuddling, being talked with, and being provided with play objects that they can look at and listen to. Giving them mobiles to view as they lie in their cribs and providing music will be beneficial. But the important ingredient is consistent nurturing through affectionate personal and human contacts. Improvement of weight condition and stature come slowly, as does return of appetite, but the vomiting and irritability responds rather rapidly to appropriate care.

With the change in infant appearance and activity, many mothers are able to feel pleasure and see for themselves that they are functioning successfully as mothers. With this comes greater self-confidence in mothering ability. The basic problems in the family structure should be clarified and modified wherever possible. This may require the assistance of a family service or other social work agencies. One cannot tell women to love their babies, but one can discuss with them the importance of affectionate experiences developmentally not only to infants but to parents as well.

The pediatrician, by being non-judgmental and encouraging, friendly and supportive of a mother in her attempts to change her mothering personality, may set an example of importance. As he takes some of the responsibility for the care of the infant, encourages her to talk about herself, her past experiences, her feelings about the baby, a mother usually responds with greater willingness to try to change her attitudes and child care practices. Such women need regular and sustained help throughout the period of infancy and the pre-school period.

If mothers are mentally sick, the infant must be placed in the care of other competent persons. This may be done by the use of a homemaker, the use of a relative as a mother substitute, or by removing the baby from his home. This last step must be done with caution, because the failure-to-thrive syndrome is not infrequently found in babies reared in institutions or in a series of foster homes. Long-lasting mental illness, autism (see page 211), or even inability in later life to put trust in oneself and others, may be the pathologic results from inadequate care in infancy and early childhood which is impersonal, unsatisfying and not in keeping with the developmental needs of the baby.

Minor variations of the failure-to-thrive syndrome are seen in babies whose weight gain and growth is satisfactory but who are chronically irritable, excessively fearful, are finicky eaters, or have frequent upsets with what the mother calls "colic." A study of these babies and their families reveals a variety of reasons for the behavior. Often the mother is unduly worried and oversolicitous about the baby's state of health and attempts to make him into something that he is unable to or unwilling to become. This is seen as she forces food into him.

Sometimes a mother and father are content with the baby, but others in the family, such as grandparents, may be pressing the parents to do things "to improve him" which are contraindicated and even harmful. The following of folklore and folk medicine falls into this category occasionally. In this instance the pediatrician must take a firm stand on the side of the parents; help them to feel they can be responsible and effective and help them affirm this so that grandparents will desist in their effort to control the baby and his parents.

Occasionally parents who have had the misfortune of experiencing illness with older children expect a repetition in the new baby. This anxiety leads them to overcare and overprotect him. Whatever the reasons, the pediatrician can help such parents as he conducts a thorough physical examination and patiently advises them on physical health problems which may be present. Without going into long psychiatric interviews, enough of a psychologic history should be obtained which gives him some idea of the nature of the family climate, the role of the parents and other persons in the care of the child.

In an informal and permissive way, a pediatrician can show his interest in the parents, particularly the mother, by non-directive and non-threatening questions. Without judgmental pronouncements, he can give guidance which is meaningful and practical. Probably more important than anything else is the mother's feeling that the physician appreciates what she is going through, and how difficult her problems are. Sometimes a didactic approach is needed to explain developmental needs and to make specific suggestions for handling a particular problem. Often such plans are best made with both parents present.

A Case of Failure to Thrive: Henry S., 6 months old

A scrawny, frail, undernourished baby had been hospitalized twice previously for periodic episodes of vomiting, diarrhea, poor sleep and a more or less constant irritability. Weight gain had been irregular and never up to normal. On this admission he was less than the third percentile in weight, and under the twenty-fifth percentile for height.

He was responsive to people by being suspiciously observant and ever-watching, but not smiling and not cuddly to hold. Examinations were made following the schema for diagnosing failure to thrive. The impression was reached that no neurologic or metabolic disease existed to explain the baby's abnormal condition. The search then for psychologic causes continued.

The parents were interviewed singly and together, and observed when they visited Henry. Mrs. S. was a thin, tired and frustrated young woman who had a limited repertoire for dealing with her infant. He had been small at birth, with a small head, hemangiomata of the face, and neck, and an umbilical hernia. She considered him fragile and she feared touching him. Part of her apprehension stemmed from the fact that she had had a series of miscarriages before, and severe phlebitis during the second pregnancy. Henry was the third baby and was not wanted. The parents had been told not to have any pregnancy so soon after the second.

On coming home from the hospital 5 days after birth, Henry had vomited often and seemed to resist the mother's feeding him. She found it fatiguing to comfort him, and became anxious, tense and unable to sleep. As her tension mounted, Henry's irritability increased. The father took limited interest in all of the family life. Being a truck driver he was away from home 4 nights a week. When present, he preferred to sleep or look at television.

Treatment in Hospital. Present hospitalization lasted 18 days. The mother seemed to gain a sense of competence as she shared her concerns with the medical staff who were interested and noncritical, who found her a rather pleasant woman despite their first impressions of her. Mrs. S. was not jealous of the staff's success in feeding the baby, particularly since after only a few days in residence he had begun to eat with greater appetite, had ceased to vomit, and had slept well between feedings.

Discussion. The mother reported that she was now sleeping better and had even gone out with her husband for two social events. After 14 days, Henry had gained 9 ounces in weight, and this seemed to reassure the mother that he was basically healthy and had the potential for normal development. Not only did his interest in food return, but by the time he was ready to return home he was smiling, grasped to reach bright colored toys, and made cooing sounds with his voice.

Modified Schema for Failure to Thrive (Idiopathic)

This diagnosis should be made only after a reasonable investigation has failed to demonstrate a more defined clinical category. While it is improper to set up "routines," the following Modified Schema of Ira K. Brandt, M.D. is suggested as a minimum study. The items are not listed in order of importance.

1. A thorough family history, especially re dwarfism, Rubella, and consanguinity, child care practices and social status.
2. Calculation of caloric intake: 3-day dietary history with breakdown as to protein, carbohydrate and fat.
3. A thorough physical examination should include: measurements of head span and circumference, chest circumference (at the xyphoid level) and abdomen at the umbilical level. The upper to lower segment ratio and the span-to-height ratio should also be determined.

    Dermatoglyphic patterns should be noted, the head should be "candled" (if a young infant), an adequate funduscopic examination should be performed, and blood pressure should be determined in upper and lower extremities.

    Complete neurologic examination.

    Developmental assessment.

4. Laboratory tests:
   a. Hemoglobin, hematocrit, white blood count and differential, ESR, PPD, VDRL.
   b. Urinalysis for routine, "Genetics Screening" and culture. The pH and specific gravity are particularly important; a urinalysis cannot be significantly negative unless the sample is acid and has a sp. gr. of 1.025 or more.
   c. The serum sodium, potassium, chloride, bicarbonate, carotene, calcium, phosphorus, phosphatase, FBS, BUN, creatinine, PBI, total protein and electrophoresis, virus anti-bodies (Rubella and CID).
   d. IVP as indicated.
   e. If mental retardation or multiple anomalies are present, chromosome analysis is indicated.
   f. X-ray examination for bone age, lateral skull, and chest.
   g. Sweat electrolyte concentration.
   h. Stool for microscopic fat, ova and parasites, pH (several).
   i. Combined ACTH and methopyrapone test (older children).
   j. F.S.H. (older children).
5. Consultation with Social Service workers and psychiatrist.

Colic

A syndrome commonly called colic may appear any time in the first several months of life although it seems to have a tendency to disappear after 4 months. It may manifest itself first in the newborn period as varying degrees of irritability of varying duration, interrupted sleep and prolonged periods of wakefulness. Crying is prominent, as is a posture with the knees drawn up against the abdomen. Flatus is frequently passed and although this seems to give some comfort, most parents complain that nothing is effective in soothing the infant.

Many etiologic factors are claimed to be involved, but for our purposes we will only discuss the psychologic determinants. In any list of causes of colic, this group seems to be almost always present. In essence it implies that a mother suffering from fatigue, family tension, and stresses arising in marriage and relationships with other people transmits her feelings and state of emotions to the baby. It is as if the baby senses her tension and fatigue, not only in the process of being handled by her, but by merely being in her presence, and responding to her manner, voice and general attitude. Therapy is accomplished by treating the mother and modifying her way of handling the baby. Anything to relieve her disquiet will benefit the baby. Since these babies frequently cry during the bath, this should be omitted certain days or reduced to a few minutes in duration. There is no need to change the food or the schedule, although the manner of feeding patiently and without tension is most important. Households in which there is much noise at sleeptime should reduce the responsible activities. Rarely is a sedative drug indicated. Separation of the mother and baby for part of every day, or even for a few days, permitting the former to get rest and relaxation may break the circle, stop the contagion of tension in the family and bring about a new understanding between both parties.

Speech Problems

From cooing and prattling, infants advance to the use of one or two words, usually in names for parents or a particularly important play object or toy. As infants are talked to, they increase their vocabulary and improve their manner of speech. They also learn how to develop concepts. It is not uncommon for some stammering to come in those children who are in a hurry to express themselves, and whose thoughts come faster than their words. Either ignoring this, or admonishing them occasionally to slow down, may be the only remedy necessary. Invariably stammering of this sort disappears as a child gains control and better coordination of his thoughts and his verbal expressions.

Parents encourage the formation of words as they talk to their children. Sometimes there is overstimulation of speech as when they are goaded to talk better, to use different words and to speed up. This may lead to anxiety on the part of the child because of his desire to get words out and the fear that he will not speak well. Lisping and other infantile mannerisms may be learned and may persist when parents reinforce them by showing amusement. Stammering may be a form of withholding emotions as well as words.

Occasionally children stop talking entirely as a way of demonstrating their opposition or negativism. Muteness may be of emotional etiology although more commonly it is associated with deafness or other physical defects. An infant may be slow in learning to speak because he is not stimulated by the voice of others; a pre-school child may regress or stop speaking after an especially traumatic event as hospitalization, the birth of a sibling, the death of a parent. It may be a means of asserting power over adults. These children often begin to speak without difficulty when this defense no longer fulfills their needs. We have seen a child of 5 years, completely mute for 4 months after the birth of a sibling, begin to talk spontaneously when the mother gave her more individual attention.

Many of the speech characteristics of the young developing child are transiently deviant and responsive to changes in the environment. For example, lisping, stammering and articulatory deficiencies are normative in the child under 5 or 6 years of age. Speech therapy is not needed for stammering or the other speech impediments common in the first years of life. Most of them are best handled by indirection, by treating the child as normal, being patient and giving him time to speak and to learn.

The autistic child who lives in his own inner world will not speak until communication with others is feasible. Aphasia due to cortical lesions may be the cause of non-development of speech, as may mental deficiency.

Habit Training Difficulties

Toddlers use food substances with which they come in contact for other pleasurable purposes than just eating. They enjoy playing with their food, smearing it, fingering it. This is not done accidentally but purposely for the tactile and olefactory gratification derived from it. Smearing with foodstuff is often similar to the smearing with feces in which the same youngsters indulge, or would like to. There is a close relationship between habit training, the pressure to conform to social expectations and the pressure to modify the eating and toileting experiences which are gratifying.

When habit training is being developed successfully, that is to meet parental and societal standards, and in consonance with a child's needs and desires, children change their habits of eating and of play quite as much as their habits at the toilet. Instead of enjoying dirtiness, they seem uncomfortable because of it, even anxious, as when their fingers get dirty in play and they come to their mothers for cleaning up. Carried to an extreme, they may demand a change of clothing because it has become even slightly soiled from food or from play materials like clay or paints, which all seem as disgusting as soiling with feces. Every pre-schooler goes through a phase of fighting against becoming clean, to one of becoming obsessively clean. They progress from a time in infancy when they enjoy defecating and smearing at will, to one when there is disgust and even fear of feces, treating the stool as if it were part of their bodies, and the toilet as if it were an instrument to be both feared and used with great caution.

The reactions against infantile gratifications gradually become sublimations in the developing child. Curiosity and interest in the body and its products are transformed into curiosity about the environment and its characteristics.

Feeding Problems

Eating behavior sharply serves as a sensitive barometer of general adjustment. The disgust with feces is carried over to a disgust of food, particularly soft and mushy substances which seem to remind them by touch, and even smell, of feces and the toilet. As a consequence they may refuse many foods because of their color, odor, or physical consistency. What we see here are the child's normal repressions and defensives operating in their attempt to keep him clean, and to prevent regression to infancy with its "dirty" habits. Some children retain violent dislikes and avoidances of special foods throughout life, but the majority are more accepting of these substances after toilet training is completed.

Feeding disturbances of this kind are not due to any direct mishandling of the feeding situation but are by-products of the habit training. Where this is carried out too early and with force, the problems of feeding are greater. Where the child is given more time to become clean, messy eating will persist longer but feeding problems may be fewer as a consequence of normal psychologic repression and modification of the impulses and thoughts associated with feces.

Children with finicky attitudes toward foods which repel them are frequently compulsively clean and constipated. Play with clean "dirty" materials such as sand and water, "play dough," finger paints, dry cereal and water combinations may help sublimate the wish to be dirty, and help them take steps to cleanliness which also gratifies their needs as well as the social standards of parents. The symptoms disappear, but where repression fails or the drive for infantile gratification conflicts so strongly with the desire for control and modification of the impulses that neurotic signs develop, more intensive psychotherapy is indicated.

Toddlers should be given some freedom to deal with their food as they like. Thus they not only develop and maintain a pleasurable interest in food and eating, but develop associated motor skill and in this way an enhancement of their neurologic development. Children denied this kind of opportunity and stimulation, especially if accompanied by other sensory deprivation, not only react to eating with displeasure and anger as if fighting for their rights, but ultimately give up the fight and regress to more infantile ways of behaving.

Sustained understimulation of several months' duration even so early in life may have the total effect of interfering with the maturation of neurophysiologic systems. Speech and language development, ability to conceptualize, and comprehension of symbols for learning in reading, writing and mathematics may not take place. One of the attempted remedies for deficiencies in learning in these areas is the use of techniques whereby the child is encouraged through play to go back to types of play which he should have experienced earlier and which provide the stimulation of which he had been deprived. This encompasses, for example, letting him be messy and smeary with art materials, encouraging him to crawl and climb, as well as walk, and even to chew and suck on bottles with nipples.

Transitory feeding problems such as refusal of food, vomiting, and crying at meal times may occur when children are learning other new skills such as walking. Once the task has been successfully learned, the unsatisfactory eating behavior stops. Parents who cannot accept these temporary setbacks, but who by coercion, cajoling, or by scolding attempt to stop them, tend to make the behavior worse and longer lasting.

Infants and children are sensitive to the feelings and attitudes of parents, particularly at feeding and bedtime. Mothers who are high-strung and excitable seem to transmit these states to their babies and young children. Telling a mother to relax, or change her attitude towards the feeding, has limited value. Helping her with her own problems is a more rational approach. Giving the mother an opportunity to talk about her feelings and to express in words her attitude about her child, may give insight. Hearing her out without criticism is reassuring, even though no psychologic interpretations are given. If that is unsuccessful, possibly a substitute should relieve the mother from time to time in the feeding, at least as a trial, preferably someone like the father or another relative who is not strange. As a rule, a succession of adults caring for a baby is frustrating, confusing, and unsettling to him.

Feeding problems associated with refusal of food because its appearance or odor is offensive have been described on pages 48, 49. Infants and pre-school children who for psychologic reasons have prolonged feeding problems characterized by vomiting, anorexia or other signs, may repeat this kind of behavior in their school and adolescent years when psychologic stress is particularly great. Neuroses at these times often manifest again the patterns established early in life. This fact has relevance when one considers the pediatrician's role in mental health prophylaxis. His first opportunities in primary prevention are taken when he does everything possible in the first few years of life in helping parents and children solve the minor problems of adjustment to new experiences in eating and habit training. These measures prevent chronic patterns of psychopathology from developing.

Constipation

The pediatrician is aware of constipation which has physical or organic etiology. He may be less well informed about the psychologic and developmental causes. Physical discomfort may precede psychogenic constipation, as when babies and children suffer pain on defecation, (as for example, when a fissure of the anus exists). In order to avoid the discomfort they withhold stool. Painful defecation leads to fear of defecation and as a consequence, stool accumulates. Parents who are obsessed with regularity of evacuation of the bowels, their own as well as of the rest of the family, put pressure on the child. They make toilet training a clash of wills as when they scold, argue and urge, and then in desperation give enemas or force him to sit on the toilet until he produces stool. Invariably, the child regards all this as punishment and as a loss of autonomy. As a rule, withholding then persists because the child wilfully or unconsciously disobeys his parents. The accumulation of feces may produce no symptoms of ill health. Sometimes there is chronic abdominal pain with a variety of complications, one of the most severe of which is a chronic dilatation and stasis of the colon and rectum.

Vigorous symptomatic treatment of constipation is rarely necessary. A more rational and humane treatment consists of treating the primary physical abnormality, avoiding manipulation of the anus and rectum as much as possible and controlling the constipation by changes of diet. In addition, taking substances such as colace, neo-cultol or mineral oil by mouth make the stools loose, soft and easy to pass.

When the parents can de-emphasize the need for regularity, most children respond on their own to the stimulation of the sphincters because of the fullness of the lower bowel, and defecate. They may not always defecate in the toilet, but even defecating in the diapers is preferable to obstinate withholding.

Withholding of stool may be a reaction to an external event such as the birth of a new baby, hospitalization or any number of other conditions which the child cannot understand, and which make him anxious. He reacts to them with body "language." It is an example of a *normal reaction* of young children as they attempt to incorporate an emotionally upsetting experience into their developmental phase and deal with it consciously and unconsciously as best they can.

It is not uncommon for young children to become constipated because they refuse to defecate in the toilet. As mentioned elsewhere in discussing habit training, normal children frequently withhold stool because the retaining provides a pleasurable and agreeable sensation. Or they may withhold from the toilet in order to deposit the feces in a place and in a manner which is highly pleasurable. Feces deposited in places where the child can play with it, by smearing and even eating, satisfies his infantile interests. Sometimes they shy away from use of the toilet because they do not understand what is involved in its use. It is as if they fear giving up the stools because they fancy defecation as involving loss of part of their bodies. The flushing of the toilet to such children is frightening, not only because of the noise involved, but because the disappearance of the stool itself is disturbing. Children may retain stool for days and weeks at a time causing simple constipation to become chronic and complicated.

When parents are able to accept the fact that children do not need to have bowel movements daily, half the battle is over. And when parents further understand that sometimes children withhold deliberately for psychologic needs, which in itself is a developmental phenomenon,

5

they are more able to have an interested but relaxed attitude. This helps the children to go through this part of their development quite easily. Such children will need no special treatment, nor do parents demand any.

It is certainly worthwhile to find out a mother's ideas and the family's attitude to constipation and obedience. Some parents who are themselves constipated and say that this condition "runs in the family," cannot accept even occasional constipation, fear its consequences and pay undue attention to it. As a consequence, their pressure on the child intensifies his difficulty. Here again, dietetic management and stool softeners given by mouth are preferred over more active measures involving the parents in manipulation of the child's body.

The mother's training of a child in bowel control involves an interpersonal relationship where feelings run high in all persons concerned. For the child, defecation is often associated with fear, guilt, and with the idea of obedience. He soon understands that defecating in the toilet is a "good" deed which pleases mother; that the stool is "bad," to be regarded with disgust, not touched, and quickly thrown away. Learning bowel control means acquiring and maintaining an approved skill which is invested with feelings; this leads to emotional maturation or disharmonies which are normally mild but occasionally severe enough to cause bodily symptoms, including retention and incontinence of feces.

The success of training depends on the child's physiologic readiness, his realization that defecation is pleasurable to him and to his mother, and that by defecating in a suitable place he wins her affection and approval, but that if he does not control his evacuations he is subject to her opprobrium.

Fecal Soiling; "Psychogenic Megacolon"

Premature, coercive enforced training often produces "psychogenic constipation" and dilatation of the lower bowel and rectum known as "psychogenic megacolon." The term megacolon may be inappropriate and had best be reserved for the designation of Hirschsprung's disease or aganglionic megacolon.

Chronic constipation with accumulation of feces may distend the lower bowel greatly so that x-ray examination leads to the diagnosis of megacolon. This condition should be suspected first by a group of clinical signs. Children with chronic constipation, especially with the symptoms designated as "psychogenic megacolon" often appear tense, anxious, irritable, insecure as well as defiant, hostile and controlling. Parents frequently talk about the constant fighting they have with their children about toilet training. Mothers complain of the fecal soiling and intermittent diarrhea in a child who is chronically constipated. Such diarrhea is appropriately labeled "paradoxical." The soiling is an involuntary seepage of feces, and should be differentiated from encopresis which is a voluntary or involuntary passage of solid stool into the clothing. Like the diarrhea, liquid stool or mucous bypasses the obstructed feces which are large enough to be easily palpated through the abdomen as a mass in the sigmoid colon and leaks from the anus. Rectal examination may reveal hard or soft feces. The uninformed physician may misdiagnose it as a tumor or a neoplasm, order x-ray pictures taken, and refer to a surgeon for operation. Under no circumstances, should surgical intervention be carried out.

In talking with the mother of such a child it may be learned that she already had felt the abdominal swelling when she bathed the youngster; that her concern about the constipation is matched with that about the child's peculiar habits of defecating in standing or supine positions, and his soiling. As newborn and young babies, there was no trouble in passing stool; the syndrome of constipation and withholding had its onset months later, usually around toilet training. (This is one important distinguishing sign to rule out Hirschsprung's disease which has a neurogenic origin, and manifests itself at birth or in the first weeks of life.)

Since avoidance of the toilet and withholding of feces for many days is the complaint, it is natural for parents to treat the symptoms by use of enemas and suppositories. Manipulation of the anus upsets the child further. His resistance is fortified and the parents become infuriated. Nevertheless the time comes when the colon is so distended with feces that the child is irritable, even in pain, and the lower bowel must be emptied. This had best be done by a physician, using an enema of colace and mineral oil, followed by manual removal if necessary. When done gently, with kindly reassurance from the physician, the child feels much better, and may even be proud of having helped empty his bowels. The anxiety of the parent is lessened as well. Psychologically it is crucial to provide the child with an active role in overcoming this difficulty.

Equally important is the physiologic result. The loss of proprioception of the anal sphincters which had resulted from the impaction and over-distention of the rectum returns gradually and the child is again able to recognize the signal to defecate. If the stools are not hard, he is more willing to defecate. As a rule, this is not done in the toilet for a while, but as the child prizes his success in regular defecation, he will increasingly attempt to act in a more grown up manner in his toilet habits.

He will be helped if parents suggest use of the toilet each day, and if his tentative approach to toilet training is encouraged by the parents' words of pleasure. But use of the toilet should not be "oversold"; casualness even in the use of praise is recommended.

Once the impaction has been removed, stool softeners may be given by mouth regularly. Enemas may also be administered by persons other than the parents, if oral medication is ineffective; but saline enemas should *never* be given unless the obstruction has been removed in order to avoid chemical imbalance and shock which may result from enemas which are retained.

There is disagreement among psychiatrists and pediatricians about when and how to empty the rectum manually and as to whether these children should be first treated psychologically. Ideally, psychotherapy should come first and all anal manipulation avoided, especially in the hands of the mother. However, when the condition has reached a point where the child is physically distressed and emotionally distraught, and the parent at her wit's end, there is merit to having a skilled physician or nurse empty the rectum and colon. There is no reasonable evidence that additional emotional trauma has resulted from relieving the child of his hoarded feces when such an advanced state of bowel dysfunction has been reached and when the manual removal of stool is done skillfully, more or less comfortably, and with some attempts at explaining the procedure to the child, so he feels informed and can cooperate actively with the procedure.

Where children are fearful of evacuating because they consider it dirty, they may be helped by encouragement to engage in "dirty" play with finger paints, sand and water, mud pies, mixtures of cereal and water. As they are able to relax in their messiness, frequently they are able to relax the anal sphincter more readily when feeling the urge to defecate—and one day to use the toilet. In severely neurotic children, the medium of psychotherapy involves such messy play. When parents are neurotic and obsessed with the child's toilet habits, severe psychopathology must be suspected and psychotherapy recommended for them.

Encopresis

This is defined as the passage of stools of normal consistency under inappropriate circumstances. The stool may be deposited in the clothing, left in places around the house and even secreted with clean clothing in a drawer. Although parents may claim that the child is unaware of the passage of feces, it is actually an event not only recognized by the child but invested with his feelings. This is no overflow incontinence as in soiling, and there is no organic basis for it.

Case of Robert H.

A typical case is that of Robert H., 4 years old, the first-born to a mother who was compulsive about her own cleanlinesss and who suffered from chronic constipation like her own mother. Both mother and grandmother had high standards, were rigid and chronically depressed. When Robert was forced to go to the toilet, he defied his mother and dirtied his pants. He had been toilet "trained" by 1 year of age. The mother interpreted training as catching his stool in the pot so there were never any soiled diapers. He was "pottied" several times a day, usually simultaneously with feeding. The stools were always firm but soft. By 3 years he had begun to use the toilet when "reminded."

The problem began at 3½ years when he refused the toilet on a succession of days. He started by withholding and later began to deposit the feces in various places. When seen in the clinic, he appeared to be a boy who was well-developed and nourished, not ill but cranky. Physical examination was negative; rectal examination was done surprisingly easily, with little resistance, (possibly accepted with pleasure), and the feces were soft. In the interview his mother spent most of the time criticizing her son, as well as the arrangement of the clinic which she thought exposed her child to sick children in the waiting room. The mother wore long gloves and on questioning revealed that she always wore rubber gloves when diapering, placing on the toilet, and bathing her son. She had been separated from her husband because of sex problems and volunteered that she was "through with marriage."

The mother thought the encopresis was psychologic but showed no insight into the mechanisms of its etiology.

The pediatrician saw the mother weekly for 1 month and reexamined the child 4 weeks after the first examination. He interpreted the physical findings and reviewed the developmental characteristics of pre-school children in general, especially in terms of toilet training and the mother's role in it. Attempt was made to explore the extent to which the mother could change her attitude towards the child's toilet habits. The physician tried to give her some insight into the nature of the problems and of the meaning of the symptom. At the fourth visit she raised the question about the need of psychotherapy and accepted referral to a child guidance clinic.

Encopresis is a symptom which almost always indicates that child and parents need skilled psychiatric evaluation and treatment. A possible exception to this is the case in which the patient has only recently shown the symptom, responds quickly and lastingly to parental education and the reassurance of the pediatrician.

Soiling and encopresis may appear in school age children and adolescents, but the psychologic mechanisms involved are different from those described here. (Attention will be given to these conditions in discussions under Adolescence on page 142.)

Sleep Problems

In the second year of life, the relationship of the baby to the mother is close and intimate. Many toddlers can hardly bear to be parted from their mothers even for short periods of time. They react to every separation with great feelings, as if their mother had disappeared forever. They cry angrily and apprehensively when the mother leaves the room or the house. Falling asleep in the evening at this time of life is difficult. It is as if the baby feared that by falling asleep, the mother would leave. Such wakefulness is best regarded as a developmental feature rather than signifying something pathologic in the child or evidence of spoiling on the part of the parents.

A mother sometimes feels helpless when dealing with these kinds of sleep problems. She does not understand how this could happen when she has been so careful and considerate in caring for the baby and answering his needs. Thereupon, her first reaction is to tie herself more closely to the house and to the child, which only seems to aggravate the problem.

There are better means by which to desensitize the child to separation. Some of these techniques include the games of peek-a-boo, or losing and finding. They are particularly enjoyable to the child, and he seeks to have them repeated frequently each day. This is a means of reassuring himself that when his mother or any other object which he loves disappears, it is not lost forever.

The infant who awakens at night as if frightened, or who has trouble falling asleep, is in need of immediate comforting; when a parent responds and reassures him, the sleep problem is of short duration. After a few nights of being talked with, offered food, having the back rubbed and tucked back into bed, the baby is helped to adjust to changes in his life. Often mothers over-react with anxiety to the sleep problem and remove the baby from the crib. They hold him for long periods of time, and then put him back with reluctance or with the feeling that his quiet is only temporary. This uncertainty of feeling seems to be transmitted to the baby who immediately proves her fears. He reawakens at the touch of the bedclothing, cries and demands to be held again.

Where this sleep pattern of crying and agitation continues nightly over a period of weeks or months, parents and whole families become anxious, angry and frustrated. In such severe cases it may be best to remove the child temporarily from the parent and place him in the hands of other competent adults preferably in his own home. While the child is being cared for by another mother figure, the mother has a chance to catch up on her own rest, to talk out her concerns, and to learn new patterns of child care.

Most children go through periods of night wakefulness, night terrors, and other behavior aberrations in the daytime. This syndrome frightens parents. Yet despite its complicated etiology it more often represents normality than a psychopathologic situation, although in some cases it may be the latter. The mechanisms of this syndrome are as follows: The normal awakening of a child which is part of his developmental pattern in the age period of 12 to 30 months, comes at a time when other important events are taking place in his life, particularly habit training.

As has been mentioned before, training in eating and in use of the toilet represent major events, which are fraught with conflicts. The child has a wish to soil and yet fears to do so lest he lose the love of his parent who is training him. In the process of becoming toilet trained, clean and obedient, he makes a compromise with his instinctual needs, which do not disappear but demand gratification in other forms. These may appear as sleep or eating aberrations. For example, the child in sleep may dream about what is hapening to him in his waking hours, what is happening to his body and to his parents. What he re-experiences in sleep is pleasurable or frightening. If the latter, he awakens, cries, and is comforted with difficulty. His wish to be messy and dirty with feces leads him to messy eating and play. But when even this is repressed, it becomes transformed into fear and disgust of dirt. The price paid for cleanliness (toilet training) sometimes is high, as when phobias develop, such as fear of vacuum cleaners, of bathtub drain pipes and other apparatus which seem to swallow up people and make them disappear like the feces in the toilet bowl. Sometimes children are afraid to fall asleep lest they lose control of their bowels and defecate in bed, thus displeasing their parents and running the risk of losing their love and care. These are the innate, unverbalized drive conflicts within the child to which he reacts with wakefulness. As parents understand this process around wakefulness, they will react with less puzzlement and anxiety.

Older children sometimes admit to physicians their fantasy that a breakdown in toilet habits, such as in bed wetting and soiling, leads to dire outcomes such as they or their mothers becoming sick and going to hospital. They see a magical connection between their behavior and other unpleasant experiences. When sleep problems appear during the time of toilet training, it is best temporarily to de-emphasize such training and reduce the pressure. Almost immediately a child treated this way returns to normal sleeping habits, demonstrating that he needs more time to reconcile his infantile needs with the demands of the outside world.

As mentioned earlier sleep problems may arise coincidentally with other events like temporary separation from mother, birth of a new baby in the family, moving to a new house, occupying a new crib, or going to a hospital. All these situations are not everyday occurrences in the life of the child, and his reactions of anxiety are appropriate.

They produce greater anxiety only in special children and the circumstances for this are not always clear. Some children are more readily overwhelmed and cannot reduce anxiety. Others from early in life have a greater abundance of inborn resilience and are better able to anticipate traumatic situations. It is as if the ego unconsciously anticipates the danger, prepares for and copes with it. As a result there are no symptoms. This mechanism is demonstrated in play when the child faces a make-believe crisis, and attempts to achieve control of the situation by playing it out. Games like losing and finding his mother, or those in which he lets himself fall down so he is not hurt and then gets up again, are examples of devices they use to desensitize themselves to danger.

In other words, he does to himself what he has experienced before, or what he anticipates will be done to him. By recreating the potentially traumatic episodes or events they lose their strength and he achieves mastery and control. Angry play with dolls is another way of attacking the aggressor. Playing with the toilet bowl in which objects are flushed down by the child, gives him the feeling of mastery over his feces. This removes some of the sting of helplessness and fear of the loss which comes from imposition by forces outside himself.

Even in young children, as mentioned before, the dream is a remedial mechanism to help them adjust to upsetting and frightening events. Such mechanisms are called abreactive devices. Disturbed sleep is to be viewed not only as a symptom of psychologic stress, but as evidence of rehabilitative efforts. These unconscious attempts at self-treatment are abetted by a parent who comforts the child in a variety of ways, and permits and encourages play in which he can symbolically master situations which lie at the base of his conflicts.

In summary, wakefulness and difficulty in falling asleep are common developmental features in infants and young children. Most sleep disturbances respond favorably to measures used by parents which allay anxiety in themselves and the children. The pediatrician can prevent severe sleep problems from developing by teaching mothers the developmental facts of infancy and childhood, how to anticipate some of the problems and how to deal with them in their early phases. He can advise the mother on how to engage the child in play activities (such as mentioned above) which help him to learn new ways of coping with situations that appear dangerous and anxiety-producing.

When this does not work and when the symptoms are more complex and appear in a variety of forms unabated over time, more intensive steps are necessary. Direct psychotherapy of parents and of the child, even those as young as $2\frac{1}{2}$ and 3 years, is often necessary to help him master the trauma.

Behavioral traits which are puzzling as to origin, because they seem unrelated to current happenings in the life of the child, usually are postponed or delayed reactions to psychologic incidents, or are revivals of earlier traumatic situations, reproducing as it were the effects of an earlier trauma which overwhelmed the child's ego and left him helpless. In such cases, dealing with the immediate situation of disturbance or only with symptom removal does not alter the basic conflict. Direct psychotherapy with the child is indicated in order to reduce the influence of the earlier experience. A variety of psychiatric techniques, from psychoanalysis to behavior-therapy, involving relearning, reconditioning or desensitizing have been developed for this purpose. (See pages 197–199, Play Activity in Pediatric Practice.)

Rhythmic Body Movements; Head-banging

These are common activities of normal infants between the ages of 3 and 12 months. Head-banging is the most worrisome and annoying to parents because they fear injury. This rarely occurs, even though the head is exposed to severe and long sustained physical force. Occasionally subcutaneous hematoma develop although these may require no treatment. They seem to cause no discomfort. The self-induced pain seems satisfying but even so is a symptom of psychological difficulty.

Head- or body-rolling often precedes head-banging. These rhythmic activities take place at bedtime, on awakening, and at times of stress during the day. Although they may be transient, most of them appear regularly each night, last from 30 minutes to 3 or 4 hours, until sleep or relaxation intervenes.

Such body movements were once thought typical of the mentally deficient. While such babies may manifest them, it is more likely to appear in children who are physically healthy but who are understimulated. Left alone or unnoticed, they react in this way in order to obtain gratification. It is said to be self-induced erotic and aggressive activity which probably is a way of expressing impulsive energies that had had no adequate discharge during the day.

Treatment consists of (1) assessing the life and health of a baby, the nature of his social contacts including the attitudes of the parents; and (2) making up the deficits. Providing rhythmic stimulation, as through sound of a metronome, or through gentle body shaking by use of a rocking crib or cradle may stop the habit. Drugs are not indicated. The activities may last several months or well into the pre-school age. Occasionally they are seen even in school children as a bedtime ritual, at times of physical illness or when they are particularly fatigued. Follow-up studies suggest that these children tend to become active children, not necessarily "nervous," but prone to rhythmic activity in response to musical stimuli. Coordination of the body and the limbs is excellent.

Breath-holding Spells

Attacks in which a frightened, hurt or angered child cries vigorously for a few breaths and then holds his breathing is familiar to most pediatricians. Cyanosis, loss of consciousness and limpness follow and there may be a few jerks of the arms and legs and even periods of increased tonus of the limbs. Although these episodes are frightening to parents and to children, when they recur (and this is not unusual in some children up until 5 or 6 years of age) the spells are tolerated even though there is disquiet fostered by fear and frustration in the parent. The spells are self-limited, since the body chemistry corrects the imbalance caused by the hyperventilation.

Breath-holding spells sometimes run in families. They are invariably associated with a behavior problem, particularly characterized by stubbornness, disobedience, and aggression. Mentally retarded children are not immune. The frequency of these episodes varies from child to child, and even in the same child at different periods, ranging from once a year to several times daily. In most children the spells tend to reach a peak of frequency usually by the end of the first year of life. The newborn may rarely evince this behavior but the most common time of onset is after the age of 6 months. Parents report precipitating factors which have an element of unexpectedness and surprise, particularly frustration, fright or minor injuries.

No direct treatment is indicated, certainly not in the use of anticonvulsant drugs, even to attempt to prevent or alleviate syncope. These spells may be viewed as symptomatic behavior suggesting a problem in the parent and child relationship which can be relieved by guidance of parents in assessing the infant's tolerances and needs. Epilepsy is to be ruled out by neurologic and electroencephalograph assessments. Syncopal attacks in adults, as well as the hyperventilation syndrome, occasionally are sequelae to breath-holding attacks in infancy.

Chapter 5

THE TODDLER AND PRE-SCHOOL AGE
(Under 5 years)

THE TODDLER AND PRE-SCHOOL AGE

Tasks in Process

CHILD

To reach physiologic plateaus (motor action, toilet training).

To differentiate self and secure sense of autonomy.

To tolerate separations from mother.

To develop conceptual understandings and "ethical" values.

To master instinctual psychologic impulses (oedipal, sexual, guilt, shame).

To assimilate and handle socialization and acculturation (aggression, relationships, activities, feelings).

To learn sex distinctions.

MOTHER

To promote training, habits and physiologic progression.

To aid in family and group socialization of child.

To encourage speech and other learning.

To reinforce child's sense of autonomy and identity.

To set a model for "ethical" conduct.

To delineate male and female roles.

Acceptable Behavioral Characteristics

CHILD

Gratification from exercise of neuromotor skills.

Investigative, imitative, imaginative play.

Actions somewhat modulated by thought; memory good; animistic and original thinking.

Exercises autonomy with body (sphincter control, eating).

Feelings of dependence on mother and separation fears.

Behavior identification with parents, siblings, peers.

Learns speech for communication.

Awareness of own motives, beginnings of conscience.

Intense feelings of shame, guilt, joy, love, desire to please.

Internalized standards of "bad," "good"; beginning of reality testing.

Broader sex curiosity and differentiation.

Ambivalence towards dependence and independence.

Questions birth and death.

MOTHER

Is moderate and flexible in training.

Shows pleasure and praise for child's advances.

Encourages and participates with child in learning and in play.

Sets reasonable standards and controls.

Paces herself to child's capacities at a given time.

Consistent in own behavior, conduct and ethics.

Provides emotional reassurance to child.

Promotes peer play and guided group activity.

Reinforces child's cognition of male and female roles.

(Under 5 years)

Minimal Psychopathology

CHILD

Poor motor coordination.

Persistent speech problems (stammering, loss of words).

Timidity towards people and experiences.

Fears and night terrors.

Problems with eating, sleeping, elimination, toileting, weaning.

Irritability, crying, temper tantrums.

Partial return to infantile manners.

Inability to leave mother without panic.

Fear of strangers.

Breathholding spells.

Lack of interest in other children.

MOTHER

Premature, coercive or censuring training.

Exacting standards above child's ability to conform.

Transmits anxiety and apprehension.

Unaccepting of child's efforts; intolerant towards failures.

Over-reacts, over-protective, over-anxious.

Despondent, apathetic.

Extreme Psychopathology

CHILD

Extreme lethargy, passivity or hypermotility.

Little or no speech; non-communicative.

No response or relationship to people, symbiotic clinging to mother.

Somatic ills: vomiting, constipation, diarrhea, megacolon, rash, tics.

Autism, childhood psychosis.

Excessive enuresis, soiling, fears.

Completely infantile behavior.

Play inhibited and non-conceptualized; absence or excess of auto-erotic activity.

Obsessive-compulsive behavior; "ritual" bound mannerisms.

Impulsive destructive behavior.

MOTHER

Severely coercive and punitive.

Totally critical and rejecting.

Over-identification with or overly submissive to child.

Inability to accept child's sex; fosters opposite.

Substitutes child for spouse; sexual expression via child.

Severe repression of child's need for gratification.

Deprivation of all stimulations, freedoms and pleasures.

Extreme anger and displeasure with child.

Child assault and brutality.

Severe depression and withdrawal.

Dynamics of Normal Development

Although the seeds of autonomy were sown earlier, this period marks the great ascendancy of selfness. Being active in the learning process promotes independence. Accomplishing toilet training gives the child a feeling of self-control and convinces him that he is in charge of himself in matters like body function, which are important. He may use this new power in struggles with parents, but even through this he learns about socialization.

The attainment of selfhood, or development of the ego in psychoanalytic terms, is met with feelings of ambivalence in most parents. They want their child to be independent, autonomous, adult-like, yet mothers especially feel some sadness at "losing their baby." The struggles of separation seen earlier are intensified now. In parent as well as child there is wish both for independence and dependence.

Out of the clash of wills come problems related to such vital experiences as eating, sleeping and toileting. These were already evident earlier. Occasionally they become manifest for the first time. These are not unhealthy or abnormal, but the unexpectedness of these difficulties often is disconcerting to those who were proud of the fact that they "never had behavior problems" with their child. They react with guilt as well as with anxiety. Because of these feelings their management of the child may be helpful or may make matters worse.

For the pediatrician, this is a time when much preventive assistance may be given by counseling parents, by reassuring them, and by helping them handle the stress with greater confidence. However, the pre-school period is not all stress and strain.

The growing child tries hard to emulate and please the parents, and he is joyful and proud with his efforts. So are the parents. They enjoy seeing miniatures of themselves, especially when the attributes are positive and compare favorably when measured against other children. The pre-school child is upset when he does what he thinks his parents want him to do, yet he fails to please them. He is confused by their change of rules. What they accepted earlier, like messiness and genital play, is not tolerated now. He is expected to be quite mature, whereas his inclinations and ability are to grow gradually. He tests out people and conditions of life in general. He is not as bold or sure of himself as his parents desire, yet he is too bold and aggressive to suit them. He has fantasies, and this is considered humorous by adults, yet he is accused of lying and not telling the truth.

The pre-school period is one of great learning about many things and play is the supreme medium of learning; the "work" of the child. Curiosity and interest in learning are at high pitch, senses are keenly perceptive. There is incessant exploration into the world of things;

words are discovered, and names for everything. Pleasure is derived from naming, rhyming, echoing words for the effect this has on parents (especially 4 letter words) as well as for their sounds. From this conglomeration of activities, cognition flourishes especially if it is encouraged and guided by parents and skilled teachers in pre-schools and day care centers. Only recently have politicians, educators and parents become aware of the importance of this period of life for setting foundations of cognitive and social learning and for training in moral and ethical judgments.

It is not surprising then that at this time of life the child is filled with "problems"; mostly the normal and usual patterns of coping which cause moderate concern to parents. Occasionally, however, there are more severe conditions which make parents and other adults legitimately anxious. Even overt mental illness may be manifest now, especially autism which represents a failure of selfhood to develop, an isolation of the child from people.

The pre-school child is old enough to be dealt with directly by the non-psychiatric physician, psychiatrist, and non-medical personnel in therapy which includes use of psychologic measures. By virtue of the mother's role-responsibilities in the family, which provides more continual and intimate contact with the children, she is better able than her husband to undertake active management of any behavior problems which develop. But she must be dealt with directly too, either individually or as a member of a group.

In psychotherapy it is not unusual for the mother to be seen much more frequently and regularly than the child. Initially meeting with father, mother and child, or father and mother together, has merit in helping assess the various factors in the personalities involved which account for the problems and which need to be modified if solutions are to be found (See pages 192–193).

The most common aspects of this age group which the pediatricians must be prepared to diagnose and treat with parents and children are described below.

Problems of Sex

Though often considered as a period free of sexuality, a "time of innocence," infancy and early childhood possess erotic pleasures of their own kind. Erections of the penis are common to boys of any age, and already are manifested in the neonatal period. It is true that a full bladder may be the stimulus then, but the result seems to be pleasurable nevertheless and it does not take him long to discover other ways of self-stimulation, especially by rubbing. Parents inadvertently stimulate by diapering too tightly, or overcleaning and rubbing the genitals. Some nursemaids are known deliberately to masturbate babies and young children as a way of quieting them.

The baby or toddler does not have thought processes as adults know them. By pre-school age, however, he is beginning to have awareness of sex differences and ways of obtaining sex pleasure. Further he is consciously and unconsciously driven to gratify himself by fantasies, masturbation and sex play with others. It is difficult, even abhorrent for some parents to realize that their children under 5 years of age find the stimulation of the genitals a source of interest, excitement, comfort and pleasure.

From these attitudes spring problems, first in the parents with their anxiety, and then in the children with their shame and guilt which they readily feel in the parents. There is good clinical evidence that censure of sex explorations, as of other learning early in life, creates conflicts and inhibitions if sustained for even a short time. The child becomes "morally good," but at a price paid not so much in early childhood but in later childhood and especially in adolescence and in the adult years. The sexual pleasure of intercourse is based not only on the physical contacts and physiologic processes involved, but equally much on the fantasy and sensuous thoughts which precede, accompany and follow orgasm. These have their origin in the attitudes and experiences of parents and children long before adult sexuality is established.

The experiences of early life are buried deeply, become unconscious, but are influential in deciding the patterns of reacting to life situations, to peers, to authority figures, and to sex drives.

The pediatrician acts constructively for mental health if he helps parents accept their young children's sexual curiosity and practices as physiologically and psychologically normal. Too often he does not have this opportunity. He is approached after there is a "sex problem." The anxious parent does not understand the infant's uninhibited exploration of his genitals, or the curiosity and play focussed on the genitals of others. Exhibitionism may be considered cute, but masturbation of self or by others is forbidden. Some parents worry that such normal behavior is indicative of precocious sex development, or a life of perversions.

They should be easily reassured, but may not be if their own sex life is fraught with ignorance, fear, doubt and shame. The remembrance of their own parents' taboos makes them feel the need to perpetuate the cultural pattern, despite or because they violated their parents' code and have felt guilty ever since. It is not easily accepted by some parents that such sex curiosity and sex play is an important learning experience. Parents confuse such normal behavior with morality but instead of tactfully guiding the child into socially acceptable behavior by distraction and substitute opportunities, they censor with moral indignation any evidence that the child's private sexual activity has become public. In general, the pediatrician can counsel the parents to respect the privacy of child and adult, to provide the child with opportunities for privacy and to help the child understand that sexual play is not socially acceptable in public, though it is an expected private option.

At this period in life, the child is impressionable and much concerned about the reaction of his parents. He builds his own behavior pattern from the parental reactions, and stores them in his unconscious. The role of the pediatrician is to make sure that the child is not being unduly stimulated by parents, by nursemaids, by siblings or by baby-sitters and to try to help parents understand their own feelings about the emotional phases of growth. Talking out one's attitudes with the physician often makes the parent more comfortable and permits him to let the child go through his learning experience without interference. Some parents are able to be verbally restrained about sex activities, but their attitude of apprehension continues and this is easily communicated to the child. The old proverb is still valid, "It is not what you say, but what you do that is important."

The pre-school period then is an important one for sex education, not by verbal instruction, but in the way that parents tolerate their children's activities, listen to their questions, answer them honestly within the limits of the question and the understanding of the questioner. As in all learning the child begins with himself, with what comes natural, with what motivates him. He learns what he is ready to learn at the time that he is ready to learn it. This in part is decided by his earlier expressions and the phase of development which he has approached.

In the past, some parents felt that their children should learn about the sexual nature of life by being given lessons, or worse by exposing themselves in the nude to children so as to help them accept sex differences. Commonly this leads to harmful sexual overstimulation rather than healthy learning. It is no measure of a parent's liberality or acceptance of his own sexuality if he permits himself to treat the child in this way. In fact, his own problems of sex may be projected onto his child in the name of education, but actually he gains perverse gratification for himself.

Freud talked about the seductive activities of parents towards their children, not in terms of overt intercourse, but in the covert ways in which parents handled their children's genitals, or body surface in general. As mentioned before, repetitive stroking of the skin can be an erotic stimulus. Taking children into bed may be erotic for children as well as parents. Some parents use the children as substitute bed partners, doing this in the name of comforting the child not only when he is sick, but when he is said to suffer from a sleeping disorder.

This is not to say that the traditional romping in bed is a taboo

6

activity for parents and children. But it must be remembered, that it may be sexually stimulating, a way for children to learn about the bodies of their parents and one way to get gratification of a sexual nature. Neither does it mean that parents should conspicuously avoid being seen in the nude or in the bath. They should be aware that these activities may stimulate the child but they should not react with over-prudish modesty, or with nonchalant exhibitionism.

In order to keep stimulation of the genitals to a minimum, parents should early teach their children how to bathe themselves, especially in the region of the genitals and anus.

Even without parental forbidding boys worry about such things as the function of their apparatus, the reasons for its difference from that of girls. Girls make comparisons and also fear the worst. Those who learn about circumcision of their infant brothers, feel they have proof that they too have undergone surgical removal, but they do not comprehend the reasons. Was it a punishment for "badness"? It is uncommon for parents these days to threaten a "cutting" as punishment, but it is still a part of fantasy to boys and girls especially if masturbation has been forbidden. It is difficult to comprehend anatomic differences, and one of children's recurrent fantasies deals with genital injury. One frequent misconception of children who have been hospitalized for whatever reason is that their genitals have suffered injury.

One of our patients believed that removal of his tonsils and adenoids consisted of giving him an enema and doing something to his penis. The attachment of a holster to collect a urine specimen and a pre-operative enema were the only events remembered. Though his throat was sore he firmly believed that the operation had taken place "on my bottom." The soiling and enuresis which followed the operation in this 4½ year old boy were ended only after weeks of talking about his surgery and weeks of playing games with toys in which he corrected his misconceptions. His parents answered his innumerable questions with the real facts. Possibly if they had better prepared him for this operation, the psychologic results would have been different.

Since the pre-school child is so vulnerable to anxiety regarding his sex organs and behavior, it is important that manipulation of the genitals and anus be kept to a minimum and that all children be told simple truths within their age comprehension about what is taking place. Circumcision had best be done in the newborn period, or after 5 years, when the child is better able to comprehend and less prone to distort.

Peer Group Socialization

As the child learns to please his parents with improved eating habits and a dry bed he is considered ready by society to join his peers in the outside world. This may be through play in the neighborhood or in a day care center or nursery school.

The time when a child is ready for group experience is usually decided more by chance than by careful decision. If he has siblings he will have been engaged in group play often, first as a passive subject then as a minor but active participant. Invariably there are at least a few children of similar age in the neighborhood, who play under the direction of one mother serving her turn as a communal baby sitter. But the federal program called Headstart has given such an impetus to the nursery school and day care center movement that many mothers now seek such a community resource for the children of 3 to 5 years of age.

The 2 year old has a limited tolerance for group relationships. He is more comfortable with one or two others at a time, for part time each day. But by 3 years he can more easily cope with a group of several peers and with one or two adults, for 3 to 6 hours a day away from home. He may experience separation anxiety at first; or the mother may feel this quite acutely since entrance to nursery school marks another milestone along the road of independence. Some parents can take such separation easily, some too readily; others tend to hold the child back. The latter need help in finding substitute gratification in other activities, especially in establishing new ties to other people. The pediatrician can suggest part-time activity or work outside of the household without implying that the modern woman "needs freedom from the tyranny of the home," or that she is fulfilled only when she has a career.

Many mothers do not need such encouragement. They feel the need to be free of the "shackles of parenthood." Such women may push their children into independence before they are ready, and reap a variety of problems which stem from overstimulation and overexpectation of achievement.

Children may regress under such pressure; speech becomes a stammer, sleep is broken by nightmares and enuresis, the child is irritable when awake, clings to his mother when she tries to leave him, has frequent temper outbursts. He is hyperaggressive, and may deliberately try to hurt and destroy. He is holding on to what he treasures. It demonstrates that he has developed thinking to a point where feeling is related to action. The first psychosomatic symptoms appear with vomiting or complaints of pain, and the child may even become feverish after crying for long periods of time. Breath holding with unconsciousness is not rare. Interpretation of the developmental nature of the child, of his patterns of evolving and of coping should be provided the parents. It may be necessary for them not only to give up the pressure, but to limit their activities outside the home. The symptoms just mentioned along with others may appear as transitory phenomena when a child

enters nursery school or elementary school. They disappear spontaneously in a few days as the child becomes familiar with the new setting,
as a mother encourages him to try to enjoy it, and if she neither pushes
him out or holds him back. When a mother spends a brief time each
day in the new school, a child feels assured of her presence and protection. As she decreases her time there, he becomes more desensitized
and able to be on his own.

Peer group association is important because it provides many learning
opportunities; how to respond to another adult, how to become a
member of a group, how to become a leader, how to deal with approval
and disapproval from others, and how to understand the feelings of
others.

Most groups lend themselves to special play, and one learns how to
share, to obey rules, to take defeat. Play materials are often more
abundant and more varied in a group. The importance of *guided* play
needs a special emphasis, because there is much evidence to show that
later school learning in academic subjects like reading, writing and
mathematics is based on the kind of experience a child has in the
under-5 years.

Play which involves use of small muscles favors writing development.
Games which make use of symbols are a foundation for learning to read.
Crawling, climbing, running help coordination. Large muscle use in
body movement helps the child get a feeling of self in mastery of
situations as well as of his own body parts. Play in making music gives
one the feeling of rhythm as well as the pleasure of doing something
successfully with others. Stimulation of all sense organs aids perception
and the capacity to use alternate and composite ways of learning. All
of these curricular considerations in the prekindergarten school enable
the child to increase his flexibility in perceiving, coping and adapting
to the multiple demands of his own needs and those of his family, community and society.

Much of the remedial work with poor achievers in school, especially
those understimulated previously or those who are physically impaired
as the brain-damaged, aphasic and autistic relies on replicating those
activities and experiences just mentioned. Deprivation of the use of
muscles, large and small, in the infancy and pre-school periods has early
effect on the emotional development of the child and if prolonged, such
movement restriction has profound effects later in life. An abnormal
motility pattern, as detected by a developmental examination, is an
important sign of an emotional deprivation in the past. Therefore appropriate preventive action is important. For example, a child whose
activity is restricted by a cast, splints or traction should be provided
with opportunities affording substitute experiences. If a child cannot
run, climb or cling, his hands should have other choices as in self-

feeding, crayoning, squeezing balls or playing with clay, throwing objects, tearing paper.

Although it is a well-known fact in pediatrics that the pre-school child is subject to many upper respiratory infections, induced by contacts with groups of people, nursery schools or day care centers are not contraindicated for most children. Attendance is taboo only in times of epidemics. In our experience, even children with cystic fibrosis, where the danger of respiratory infection is particularly great, usually tolerate quite well the physical health risks involved in joining a good nursery school because they gain much emotionally and socially. Such physically sick children frequently are too isolated, too much reared in artificial environments so they are deprived of opportunities to learn many things.

Whenever possible we have found it beneficial to consider the needs of the whole child, in arranging his activities in the home and outside. We believe that for most children, with whatever chronic disease, some kind of nursery school program is indicated. It may be that special groups should be arranged, with smaller numbers of children, with more adults, and with a physical plant which is particularly arranged to make it less threatening to the physical health of the child.

Obviously, all nursery schools cannot become special treatment centers. But diversity of school and curricula are possible and desirable. Even schools for normal children may be able to cope with a few who have special needs. Each school should have a medical consultant who is readily available, not only to advise about individual children, but to meet with the staff periodically, and with the parents to make plans for the entire organization. The federal program Headstart suggests medical supervision on a regular basis to provide physical examinations, follow-up treatment, attention to the physical plant, aid in planning meals (if these are provided), and consultation for emergencies. The sharing of information by teachers and physicians, along with nurses and social workers, does much not only to improve the educational atmosphere of the school, but to enhance care in the home.

Feeling, Fantasy, Reality

Life begins as a pragmatic experience. As described before, the new-born derives pleasure from the care he receives—feeding, cuddling and comforting—without knowing the circumstances which provide him with what he needs. He takes life for granted, is gratified by what is pleasurable and feels pain when he is unsatisfied.

Although he sees objects outside of himself, he does not perceive them as separate. Going through a series of steps, in the next several years he develops the sense of space, time and causality, and engages in processes which help him distinguish other objects from himself.

In the latter part of the pre-school period, the child can act on experience and with some foresight because sensations and perceptions have been collected and stored as memory traces. His thinking is not yet rational and conceptual, however. Progress in this direction comes through learning by play, especially in symbolic activity, make-believe play, by verbal reasoning and the increased capacity of memory. Sometimes his play is upsetting to parents who view it as deliberate distortion of the truth, or as fantasy bordering on the bizarre, hence characteristic of mental illness.

A child who states that an object with which he is playing is something else is usually aware of his misrepresentation and his sense of reality is not in question. But sometimes when he relives the past in a way that is more acceptable than it had been at the time, as when a fearsome animal is viewed as friendly, he may not be aware of what he is doing. In essence he is unconsciously desensitizing himself to a fear. He is able in other situations to recognize the real and the imagined. In other words reality testing has not broken down and he is not mentally ill. When he plays out scenes of jealousy, or when he dreams in sleep, he is trying to assimilate experiences which in the daytime were repressed because they were painful and consciously he no longer remembers. When parents complain about the nightmares and the fantasies in play, they do not realize that these are all important mechanisms of self-repair, of mastering anxiety and of integrating vicariously and repetitively experiences that were too difficult to assimilate when they occurred.

The child under 5 years of age plays the role of older persons, siblings and especially parents. He is trying out his future role, especially now when his conception of maleness and femaleness is blurred. Sex differences are experimented with in games of fantasy as children dress in clothing of their own and the other sex. This should not frighten parents and they should not consider this as evidence of pre-ordained sex perversion or transvestism. The game of dressing up gives children the opportunity of imagining themselves in the role of fathers, mother, brothers and sisters.

Girls may play tomboyish games and even dress in boys' clothing as a way of experiencing masculine strivings. Such behavior is not sexually deviant particularly when it is accompanied by interest and pleasure in feminine strivings. Dressing like a boy serves the purpose of providing imitation and identification with boys and thus is something of a defense against envy and rivalry.

It is less common for boys to dress like girls, since our culture already in the pre-school period lets boys know that the masculine role is more highly esteemed. If boys of 5 years or older continually prefer female clothing, express the wish to be a girl, adopt a girl's name, play with dolls, the physician should consider psychiatric consultation for the child. One pattern in such deviant development involves an abnormal mother-son relationship and may be based on a maternal role which is dominant either because there is no father, or he is too passive to be involved with his child's life. It may indicate that the mother has a deviant personality; that she is trying to gratify herself sexually through her son instead of with her husband. Some mothers openly prefer that their boy be a girl; some use him as a replacement for a female child who was never born or who died; or the boy represents an elder or younger sister to whom the mother was unusually attached and is attempting to recreate in the person of her son. Such maternal rearing may cause transvestism in the boy.

The pre-school period is recognized as one with many conflicts between child and parents. The Oedipus Complex has been formulated as an explanation for the child's struggles with them as he attempts to define his own sex role. The boy wishes not only to be like the father, but *to be* the father. He courts the love and attention of his mother. Jealousy and envy of the father is shown in outbursts of anger, rebellion against him, make-believe play and fantasies in which it is evident that the father is the target of hateful and destructive wishes. Parents are upset by this behavior, and so is the child, who fears retaliation.

A vacillating independence is characteristic of this age also. The child wants to be independent of the mother but becomes dependent when in need of comforting. The ambivalence is dissatisfying to him and puzzling to the parents. If the father can withdraw gracefully from the struggles which his son originates, show affection and interest in him despite his behavior, be patient but firm as a father and resolute as a husband, and if the mother can remain loving but not the lover of her son, time will be on the side of all parties concerned.

The normal resolution of the Oedipus Complex comes when the boy makes a comfortable identification with the father, is proud of the affiliation and takes on some of the attitudes of his manliness. Where the father is absent by death, divorce and so on, the lack of a rival may cause anxiety as when the boy reacts with a fantasy that the father has been removed by the mother as punishment for his masculine aggression. As a result, feelings of manliness are experienced as uncomfortable and are difficult to attain.

The girl also suffers from rivalry with her mother. She tries to be exclusively important like a wife to her father as she cultivates seductive attitudes towards him. She struggles with ambivalent feelings around independence from her mother whom she still needs and loves but tries to do without. In play she recreates scenes in which she tries to cope with her feelings. Fantasies of jealousy as well as outright expressions of hatred for the mother are hard to accept with equanimity by the mother, who has given affection and understanding care. But this trying situation is also resolved in time as the little girl identifies with the mother and as the latter is comfortable with her role as mother and wife, feeling no need to compete with or to subjugate the daughter.

In play the little girl pretends to be a woman like her mother, performing domestic chores and mothering and the boy plays as a doer, emulating the father's activities. To cope with their ambivalent feelings of hatred and affection for parents, children may daydream that they are orphans or that these are not their "real" parents but hateful interlopers.

Children can distort reality to fit such unconscious fantasies. A child under 5 years of age is able to some degree to tell the difference between reality and fantasy, but increased accommodation of reality comes about only with the development of intuitive thinking after 5 years. Then the child is increasingly aware of discrepancies between his judgments or pretenses about the way objects will behave, and what he observes to be the realities of their actual behavior. He may attribute living qualities to inanimate objects, a trait called animism. The continual wearing down of false beliefs by facts of reality lead to correct judgments and operational thinking. While the child does this himself, he is aided by teachers and parents who answer his questions accurately and honestly. This is not to suggest that they try to end his imagination which serves creative as well as recreational purposes. The development of speech, permitting the verbalization of perceptions of the world assists reality testing. It allows for sharing of experiences through communication. This is important for learning of every kind.

When a child undergoes severe stress as when he is separated from parents by hospitalization or by death, and when his parents cannot give him the affection and attention he needs, he regresses. In one form this may appear as inability to test reality appropriately for his age, when fantasy as urgent wishful thinking may appear as lying.

When faced with experiences it cannot master at once, an immature ego attempts to find part solutions and fears develop. The commonest of these experiences are trying ordeals in the doctor's office or elsewhere, knowledge of a death or injury, violence in a TV program, sexual stimulation, disapproval from teachers, thunder and lightning, quarreling of parents, etc. A child may appear to take such experiences quite casually during his waking hours, but the lingering fears connected with them are often asserted at night time in bad dreams or anxious wakefulness. The fears may be expressed in fantasies in a sort of magical thinking to explain the phenomena. As the child's experiences are reconstituted favorably, his memory and reality testing become better developed; intelligence and logic replace primitive thinking and the fears vanish.

Parents ask at what age and stage of development lying is normal and when distortion of truth should end. It is obvious from what has been said before, that reality (truth) is arrived at by means of stages. At first fantasy is acceptable but truthfulness is appreciated. Wishful thinking dominates because it provides safety and pleasure. This is part of the primary process of mental functioning. As children grow, their ego development lays the foundation for ability to make distinctions between one's imagination, one's body and external reality. They become aware of their needs and acts which satisfy or control those needs as differentiated from the expectations and acceptable behavior held by the family and community.

Some children take longer to develop their ego functions and continue to lie, innocently unaware of their distortions. All children (even adults) regress to fantasy-lying when faced with excessive frustrations and disappointments. They use these means for coping with pain by substituting wishful pleasure. All children, like adults, have the capacity also when their ego maturity is advanced, to deny the truth in order to gain material advantages and to escape punishment. Possibly this distortion of the truth is more truly lying because it represents a form of delinquency. Human beings seem to be mixtures of "innocent lying," fantasy lying and delinquent lying. Sometimes it is not easy to disentangle these, and with the change in the mores of our society it appears that more and more of the delinquent lying is found acceptable as "innocent lying." But we should be sobered by the knowledge that developmentally, innocent lying is representative of weak ego control, regression, and infantilism in general.

Conscience

At the end of the pre-school period (4 to 6 years), the child shows by his words, acts and dreams that he has developed mechanisms of moral and ethical judgment. It does not mean that he always knows what he should do, or is able to do what he should. His ordering of values is not perfect but he does realize that decision-making involves a consideration of many alternatives and the ability to project the consequences of the various alternatives. Even at this age, he is aware that guilt goes hand in hand with decision-making when there are alternatives.

By 5 years of age he shows that he has a conscience which makes him critical of himself and serves as a censor and punisher. In psychoanalytic terms, the conscience is the conscious part of the superego, which is a structure crystallized from the ego during resolution of the Oedipus Complex. Saying this differently, it means that babies feel pleasure or unpleasure by the way they are cared for, and it does not take long for them to consider those persons who provide pleasure as

good, and the others as bad. Already in the first year, they learn that
there are certain things disapproved of by the parents; they learn
not to do them in order to earn love and avoid punishment or shaming.
As they grow, infants identify with the persons who take care of them
and who teach them. By imitation they take on those values, habits and
mannerisms. As the boy identifies with his father and the girl with her
mother, they not only resolve the Oedipal conflict, they also crystallize
their own inner voice of values and conscience. This enables them to
replace gradually the parental voices of right and wrong with their own
self-directed and guiding voice of approval and disapproval in social
behavior.

Parental discipline becomes built into the control the child has over
his own activity. He takes on the prevailing attitudes around him, as to
what is good and bad, and learns what society's representatives teach
him.

Conscience development depends not only on the way the child receives the demands of his parents, but how he perceives them. If a
child has been in a good general relationship with his parents, he tries
to be like them. This means taking on their ideals, whatever they are,
and applying them to the external as well as the internal world. From
this develops the child's *"ideal self."* In a way, it is as if he feels at
one with the parent, and symbolically re-establishes the unity between
himself and his mother which was so symbiotic at the beginning of life.

If the child has been in an unresolved conflictual situation with a parent during the early training years, the child will ignore or rebel further.
The parent interprets this as opposition and stubbornness. He may
deliberately not do what his parents wish him to do, as in the matter of
becoming toilet trained. Or another mechanism may be invoked
unconsciously, that of reaction formation (opposing the infantile impulse
with its opposite). During the phase of sphincter control and becoming
self-assertive, all infants develop the psychologic mechanisms of reaction
formation which further regulate general behavior.

Reaction formations are attitudes which are diametrically opposed to
forbidden impulses and activities, especially the sexual and aggressive
ones, and appear as use of "good words," clean behavior and kindly
attitudes. All these characteristics please the parent. The child shows
that he has fashioned himself after the adults whom he loves and fears
to offend. His internalization of parental wishes and attributes is reinforced by their praise. He learns to express and to feel shame, disgust,
pity and compassion in accordance with social expectations. But in this
process of "growing up," he does not give up completely the opposites
of these traits. The "bad" impulses being repressed, remain in the
unconscious but break out occasionally in symptoms, as when a child
regresses to infantile behavior under stress, or when he is mentally sick.

The final shaping up of the conscience comes between 3 and 6 years when the boy and girl renounce their feelings of hostility and rivalry toward the parents. This resolution of the Oedipus Complex through identification with the parent of the same sex represents the child's taking over control of his own impulses by "internalizing the parents," by developing his own evaluating system and his own overseer of thoughts, words and actions. The conscience, or superego, is a judge, and the source of self-condemnation and hatred, but also of self-approval, self-esteem and good behavior. It exercises constant surveillance over conscious and unconscious impulses and conflicts. It can be a healthy regulating mechanism or unhealthy, and in the latter instance produces a severely inhibited, distorted, or undisciplined personality.

Overstrict Conscience

In childhood these may appear as compulsions where a child actually punishes himself by performing acts or thinking obsessional thoughts which interfere with his engaging in forbidden pleasures and activity as when he is preoccupied with conflicts about dirt and cleanliness, fecal contamination and sexual fantasy. Examples would be children who are so busy washing their hands, and being dressed in clean clothes, that they are unable to play. Others demand bathing after having a bowel movement, or resist going to the toilet entirely lest they soil themselves. (See pages 50 to 56 for notes on problems of toilet training.) Other compulsions may lead a child to an unusual dependent clinging to a mother, or a fear of leaving her which are mechanisms for warding off destructive wishes and feelings towards the mother. This may be manifested also by a child who, when away from home, talks about the dangers to the home and the people in it; who speaks of fear of having the house burn down, and whose fears are confirmed whenever he hears a fire siren.

Children develop ritualistic mannerisms as protective devices. Frequent body cleansing is one of these. Others may be tics and habit spasms. Some children are afraid to look at certain people, lest their thoughts have magic powers and something bad happen. Watching a cripple is interpreted as a threat to their own body intactness. They may squint as if trying to shut out visions of something distasteful and fearful. (For further discussion of such phenomena see pages 131 to 133.)

The voice of conscience stems from fear, although it may also come from affectionate approval, as when the child has respect and trust for the parent. Guilt is a common and prominent emotion felt when the conscience works to keep a person morally and ethically straight. Anxiety expressed directly or in the guise of symptoms is also a common concomitant, as mentioned before. Guilt and anxiety in themselves are not all bad or harmful; they are essential as are frustration and conflict for the growth of adaptive capacities and realistic organization of the personality.

What makes anxiety and guilt *pathological* is the degree in which they manifest themselves, their duration, the time of their appearance in the life and experiences of a particular child, the appropriateness of the parental standards against which the child is measuring himself, and finally the toll they take in the form of incapacitating symptoms.

The conscience is not infallible. Sometimes it reflects parental distortions, as when like the parental conscience, it overemphasizes the importance of certain acts and is unjustly critical. This induces a superabundance of guilt which overwhelms the child with negative feelings. The fallibility of a conscience is also shown when it distorts parental standards which are too lax, as when parents are unable or unwilling to limit their child's behavior, and show him no standards of conduct. This implies that he need have no feelings of responsibility towards other persons. The conscience which children assume and fashion after such delinquent parents, or learn from other adults, may be defective in being unusually harsh, or ineffective and even relatively non-existent.

The pediatrician is not afforded opportunity to directly help a child develop his conscience. His contacts are too infrequent and the relationship is too often limited to activities dealing with pain and the stress of sickness. However, the physician appears (or should appear) as a model of deportment, a mature individual who is compassionate, tolerant and yet disciplined. With the young child, he serves best through the parents as he helps them with their problems of setting standards, establishing limits of conduct and fashioning methods of discipline. By interpreting the needs and behavior of children and the proper roles of parents during infancy and early childhood, the physician can make parents aware of the nuances of child care which have psychologic significance for conscience development. In helping parents with their own distortions of conscience he can indirectly foster a more healthy one in the child. This is important mental health prophylaxis, and a role which the pediatrician can perform naturally.

With the older child and especially the adolescent, the physician's influence is directly on the child. By design, but more often by chance, he provides a model as he uses his own moral and ethical judgment in dealing with the child in a variety of crisis situations. For example, when he is honest in explaining what he is going to do to the child, especially when this is painful, he promotes trust. When he has respect for the feelings of child and parents, and permits them to be together in hospital so that the mother is available for comfort and support, he combines compassion with moral and ethical decision-making. When a physician helps a child face grief, he demonstrates clearly his own views of life and death. Where the physician is consulted about matters of behavior and conduct, he complements, reinforces and even substitutes the standards and values of parents. He can approve or disapprove of his patient's behavior without a rejecting or punitive attitude. But like the conscience of parents, the physician's conscience and judgment are also not infallible. This being so, the role of the judge is best not assumed when one is trying to help a patient with conduct problems. It is safer and more effective to use techniques which help the patient appraise a situation and come to his own decision as to the relevance, moral and ethical stance of his acts. (See Therapeutic Management, Chapter 9).

Aggression

The term aggression commonly means behavior that is intended to attack something or someone. All persons act aggressively on occasion, using a variety of approaches befitting their developmental ages and their states of emotional health.

The infant's aggression is used indiscriminately and destructively. It is tamed and controlled by mechanisms within himself as he learns to cope with the demands of persons training him. His aggressive impulses become sublimated into culturally acceptable behavior as environmental control called socialization acts as an influence towards helping develop internal control.

The infant's aggression is primitively expressed as rage, leveled against himself as well as others. As he grows he increases his repertory of acts of aggression and learns both how to use them more subtly as well as how to control them.

The toddler's attitude towards the world is ambivalent. He swings between feelings of love and hate, acceptance and rejection, passivity and aggression. All of this is shown in his reactions to toilet and other training. Aggression is one of the high points of that period of life and it is shown in half playful, provoking attitudes towards the mother who is attempting to teach him various habits of eating and toilet training. If a child is emotionally upset at this time, the aggression becomes more destructive, more hostile and may be turned against himself as well as against other persons and inanimate objects.

In violent temper tantrums, episodes of head-banging, or biting of self, he shows that the aggression is directed against himself and uncontrolled. He may even be difficult to control externally by parents and other adults. Not only does unbridled aggression frighten the child, but fear may be an underlying cause for its expression. When overt aggression is absent, one suspects that this is repressed and will manifest itself in some other way. Unaggressiveness is an indicator of bygone conflicts which still exact a price. (See page 86 on Passivity.)

Some of the noisy, negativistic and angry behavior which young children show towards their parents is sometimes mistaken for behavior aimed to hurt, although it may not have such aims. By strict definition of the term such behavior therefore does not invariably qualify as aggressive. Self-assertion is not to be confused with aggression.

People differ considerably in the way they perceive an aggressive intent in the behavior of others. Parents usually view aggression as containing elements of hostility and they do not approve because of the disrupting influence it may have on the lives of others. It is a frequent complaint of parents who come to the physician for advice on how to manage it. The presenting complaints usually are the following: unmanageableness, temper tantrums, naughtiness, disobedience, spitting out food in anger, spitefulness, overactivity, constant screaming, destructiveness and cruelty.

Often in a routine visit, a mother asks, "How do I handle my child when he strikes me?" or, "What can I do to stop fighting?" "When do I try to stop it?" In this era of permissiveness, many parents still ask about limiting aggression. A direct answer is that aggressive acts are always to be terminated when they endanger the safety of the self, or of others, and when they severely damage property. Another reason for limiting aggression is that it often produces anxiety in the child. Part of such anxiety arises from the punishment invoked, and when punishment is repeated many times through early childhood, situations that provoke aggressive feelings gradually arouse anxiety too. Another cause for such anxiety is the child's fear of no limit to the expression of the destructiveness of such aggression when it is directed against himself or those he loves the most.

Parents tend to react to aggression with counter-aggression because of their own uneasiness and discomfort; but having punished the child, parents also become anxious, guilty, embarrassed and self-depreciatory.

The child may react to his parents' discipline, and to the anxiety aroused by it, by avoiding the direct aggression toward the parents. He learns subtle substitutes, or shows aggression when away from the parents, as a displacement phenomenon. The impulse to be aggressive has not been reduced; in fact, it may have been made stronger by this evasive technique.

One way of helping children with their impulses to destroy and to be aggressive is through providing them with games and encouraging play which helps them learn how to control and how to inhibit their emotions. Children who would otherwise act out their aggression by spitting, hitting, kicking, attacking and provoking may sublimate their feelings in games of competition and use of the body in sports and physical activities. Another way of being aggressive is by talking, scolding, yelling and screaming. The young child uses these methods, but may learn how to check such excessive aggression through play involving use of the mouth for chanting, singing, and shouting. This is a healthy way of discharging aggression. Adults talk aggressively and this is a behavior of which society approves. The transformation of aggressive impulses into work and learning activities is essential for the mental health of children and adults.

It is well known that aggressive behavior by children is found unsatisfactory and unacceptable by adults. Yet in our society today we put a high premium on aggression in competing with peers in school and with colleagues in business. Processes of acculturation and socialization which began in infancy help the child learn how to be competent in the use of his aggression, to practice self-control, but emphasis is less likely to include the principle that in aggression he must harm no one. The tactics of the commonly admired professional football player come to mind in which the aim is to win at any cost, particularly through competitive aggression and disregard for injury dealt one's opponents. There is good reason for children to be confused by the different models of behavior set up for them in early childhood and later life.

Children seem to differ constitutionally in the amount of aggressiveness they are able to demonstrate. This has led some people to believe that there is a biologic determination of this trait. In assessing aggressive behavior in terms of its normality or abnormality, one should look at: (1) frequency and quantity; (2) its appropriateness for the occasion (present in situations where it is expected?); (3) the quality and form it manifests; (4) identification of the object against whom the aggression is directed, and the circumstances calling it forth.

Children who have difficulty controlling their impulses and who are described as chronically aggressive or hyperkinetic, should be appraised not only psychologically, but also by physical examinations, electroencephalograph and x-ray pictures to rule out organic brain disease. Extreme cases of impulse disorder on an organic basis are those which follow encephalitis, or brain concussion after head trauma from automobile and sled accidents or severe falls. Such children have a change of personality; from normally timid, self-contained, compliant and well-behaved children they become restless, eagerly aroused to anger, irritable, distractible, and subject to violent rages. They show severe and disorganized overactivity, a short attention span and impulsivity. Psychopharmacologic agents along with psychotherapy are recommended. Children with epilepsy may have some of these characteristics. The prognosis is guarded, and convalescence is interminably long, but the discovery of new drugs may greatly improve the outcome of many patients.

Parents whose young children are excessively aggressive frequently are fearful that this presages delinquency in later life. There is no positive correlation of that kind although many children who early are subject to such behavior tend later to show obsessional compulsive personalities, perhaps their way of taming the aggressive impulses.

It is always hoped that a child who is advanced in ego development and intelligent will have better control of his aggressive impulses. Unfortunately this is not so. Children whose psychologic development is precocious may have an increase in neurotic conflicts and symptoms. Some children may be so influenced by parental control through punishment or other means that they give up manifesting their aggressive impulses in relationship to other persons and instead become withdrawn and involved in daydreams. Such dreaming, in which one fantasies desired action is utilized by all persons and in that sense is normal. What is pathologic, is when a child becomes overly compliant, is unable or incapable of showing any negative reaction and substitutes daydreaming entirely.

Just as some children are more aggressive by nature, so parents differ in their use and tolerance of aggression. Mothers who punish their children most severely for this behavior report that their children display it more than others. Which comes first is not always clear, whether it be the child's temperament with its higher level of aggressive impulses, or the mother's attitude of intolerance which makes her punish, and leads to his counter-aggression in which the mother's behavior is used as a model. Such circularity may be broken when the physician is able to help parents modify attitudes, and to suggest other methods of discipline and play which permits sublimation of the drive.

Some parents are overpermissive of a child's impulsivity. Such a parental attitude increases the amount of aggression displayed in the home and does not decrease fantasy about it, especially when permissiveness is unnatural to the temperament of the parent and is used only because it is "modern." Children reared in over-permissive homes often seem angry. They do not get along well with peers who in turn retaliate against them. It is commonly reported by a mother that "he doesn't get along with other children and has no friends." Occasionally the child deals with parental over-permissiveness by turning excessively against aggressive behavior in himself and others, becoming constricted and moralistic. Such parents had best be advised to be less permissive of aggression leveled against them, but should not combat it with counter-aggressive punishment. Setting and upholding limits consistently (which is discipline rather than punishment) helps children learn the rules of life, even though such learning is not easy and never palatable.

Case of John A., age 5 years: Aggressive Behavior

The problems listed by his adoptive parents were "edginess, temper tantrums, short attention, bossy with friends, cruel with animals."

John had been adopted at 6 weeks, and was an only child of parents who were in their early 30's. They wanted a child to "complete" their marriage which had been happy until the mother found she could not conceive. The father worked as junior executive in an advertising agency, earned well, was moderate in his habits, enjoyed spending a few hours on Sunday afternoon with his son. He came from a large family and had been embarrassed by being childless. Mrs. A. was a housewife who "wanted to be a competent mother." She worked at this, read many books on child care and was permissive in her attitudes about eating but felt uncomfortable with John's slowness to be toilet trained. On occasion she had fought him on this by insisting that he sit on the toilet for 3 hours. She regretted this, tried to make up for it by paying no attention to his toilet training for several weeks because he had seemed angry and obstinate in eating.

In rearing John she had felt doubly responsible because she was "an adoptive mother." She could not easily limit John's naughtiness, never spanked, rarely scolded but preferred to plead and cajole, or say he owed her love and obedience because she loved him "more than anything in the world."

John had been told that he was adopted, never asked about the circumstances but in anger often remarked that he hated his mother and wanted to return to his real mother.

A tonsil and adenoid operation at 3 years of age had been difficult and marked the beginning of the present difficulties. He had been admitted to hospital without any preparation psychologically, objected to leaving his mother to go to the operating room, and when coming out of the anesthetic he had wept uncontrollably for 2 hours, in which time he had begun to bleed and had to be returned to the operating room. After 2 days in the hospital in which time he seemed unusually quiet, he returned home and there refused to eat, slept fitfully, wet the bed and soiled for the first time in 6 months.

This behavior gradually changed but the mother noticed that temper tantrums without apparent reason were common. At 3 year of age he had been admitted to a good nursery school, had trouble separating from his mother but gradually adjusted well. In the school he was considered intelligent, but overactive, mean to the other children, destructive, and tried to be the boss. He remained in the school for 2 years and at the time of coming to the pediatrician with his present problems he was about to enter the kindergarten.

Examinations. John was a well developed, robust looking and healthy child. Physical examination revealed nothing to indicate central nervous system disease. He asked many questions of the physician, wandered about the room and seemed apprehensive about needles. When forbidden to touch certain objects, he listened, but was not dissuaded from his need to touch. His mother made no attempt to interfere, but asked him to stop for her sake, and called him "lover." She seemed surprised but pleased when the physician told the boy to sit in the chair and look at a book. When the boy whined that he didn't want to do this, the physician was firm and demanded that he sit quietly. The boy accepted this and spent 5 minutes looking at the book, periodically glancing at the physician.

It was suggested that the problem seemed psychologic and would best be handled beginning with an interview at another time with both parents. The mother said it would be difficult for the father to come in, but the physician said that he felt it was important that this be arranged. A time was set 1 week later. The physician bade the boy and his mother a friendly good-by, but the child refused to return the greeting.

The father and mother came at the appointed time. The pediatrician introduced the subject by saying he knew what the problems were, but wanted the parents to discuss what they believed were the issues, and the reasons for the boy's unsatisfactory behavior. The physician said he was not sure if one or both of the parents were concerned and to what extent.

The father began to speak, saying that he did not find parenthood very satisfying but tolerated John's behavior because he rarely saw his aggressiveness, since he was better behaved when he was around. Having a child, even an adopted one, had made him feel more comfortable than he had been without one but there was still the stigma attached to the fact that the boy was not their biologic child. In disciplining, he was firm but not cruel, and like his wife he had never spanked. He did not believe it important, or pleasurable to himself or to the boy, to spend more time in recreation with him.

Mrs. A. also expressed displeasure at her inability to have a child, but said that she loved John greatly and wanted to show him this by providing a good home and showing much affection. She interpreted the latter as setting no limits, being permissive, and "never losing my temper." She did not feel that her life was empty, since she believed that a mother's primary duty was in raising children. She dreaded the time when John would be grown up, and hoped that she would have him as her young child for a long time to come.

She was asked what preparations she had made for his separating (by going to school), and what thoughts she had about her own life later on when he was old enough to leave home. Her response was that she rarely thought about this, but could consider taking foster children as replacements for John. Mr. A. did not think too well of the idea but agreed that his wife should find some substitute activity. Maybe this could be community work he said.

After 45 minutes of discussion, the father said when asked about it that he felt he had benefited by the interview but that the problem was mostly one between his wife and John. He suggested that Mrs. A. return to the physician for guidance. Arrangements were made for this.

Mrs. A. was seen 1 week later. Attempts were made to help her see the value of changing her approach to child discipline. It was recommended that she set up a more structured and limiting technique and try not to use admonition, cajoling, or pleading for reciprocity of affection. The physician tried to point out that he had set an example of limiting the boy at the first interview and that the boy had responded as if he knew what was in the physician's mind and was able to comply. There was talk of how the mother might help the child enter kindergarten; to take him there and neither desert him nor spend days on end in the school until John "adjusted."

The physician explained that it was important for her to become interested in activities other than child care. Various plans were suggested and she finally agreed to apply as a volunteer in the local hospital, department of pediatrics, as a "sitter" with sick children whose parents could not visit them. Further, the social life of the family was examined. It had become limited because of the mother's need to serve John. Mrs. A. planned to again try to activate relationships with friends which would bring her and her husband out of the home.

The issues around child adoption were discussed, with an attempt to point out how children feel about this, their fantasies regarding their biologic parents, their oedipal feelings towards their adoptive parents, as well as the parental worries about being good parents. The mother was told that there was no need for her to be "exceptionally" competent as a mother of an adopted child. At the termination of 45 minutes another appointment was made for 6 months later.

At that appointment, the mother believed that she had made

progress in weaning herself from John and permitting him to enter school with greater independence. She still tried to be a model parent but had stopped begging him to "mind" her because she loved him. She was finding pleasure in volunteer work at the hospital, as well as in the several parties she had arranged in her home. Her husband also had seemed happier, "more like his old self" as she attended social events with him. She had decided not to take any foster children and spoke with some pride and pleasure of the time when John would be grown up and on his own.

John was doing well in kindergarten. He was a leader and had learned to be less impulsive in his relationship with the other children who were no longer afraid of him. The teacher was a firm disciplinarian who said that John had first reacted to her with anger by hitting her. When she had responded by separating him from the group and giving him a chance to "play out his anger," he had soon become affectionate and more tractable. On one occasion he was found to have removed one of the guinea pigs from the cage, and was pressing it rather hard. Subsequently, he was not permitted to handle the guinea pigs except in the presence of the teacher. He was then allowed to stroke, feed, and take care of it. He had been increasingly concerned with its well-being, particularly as to who was going to feed it over a weekend. At school he had told his teacher that he was adopted, that his parents loved him and they had decided to keep him although sometimes he was "bad." He rarely talked about his father, but then only in terms of his manliness and someone that he wished to be like.

Comments. Although this child does not represent one of the aggressive, chronically angry and hostile children frequently seen in the adopted, particularly after long residence in foster homes or institutions, yet he has some of the characteristics of those who are anxious about their new relationship. This boy seemed to have difficulty understanding his adoption, and his fears about losing his parents may have been activated at the time of the tonsil and adenoid operation and his separation from them. Therapy consisted of primarily working with the mother, and helping her to rearrange her life particularly in terms of her son and her husband. Anticipatory guidance consisted of helping her look at the future and planning for it. The role of the understanding teacher was also important in directly helping John.

Passivity

As a rule parents and teachers complain less frequently about this trait than aggressivity and impulsiveness. In our society, children who are quiet, obedient, less assertive, undemanding, reserved and even shy, are considered "good." These traits are particularly expected in girls. In fact, they may be complained about only if they appear in boys, who are expected to be leaders; aggressive, competitive and "sowers of wild oats." But these characteristics may represent a pathologic condition in both boys and girls.

Children under 5 years of age, who are attempting to deal with their oedipal relationships, their death fears and wishes and their various hostilities, usually show inhibitions. These produce passivity. The normal child does not show this excessively. It will change as he moves into new phases of development, and as he deals with new stresses and uses different ways of coping.

Whether complained about or not, physicians should be concerned about babies and children who are too good, who do not protest against unfavorable external circumstances. These traits could represent organic damage of the central nervous system or a defective ego. The absence of distress or anxiety when threatened with loss of love may be the first indicator of autistic withdrawal. Children who separate too easily from parents are those who later on fail to form normal relationships. Boys who are passive, who identify more readily with women than with men, are typical of those who have for one reason or another not had an opportunity to relate to men, to see what men are like, to imitate and to try to be like them. Mothers who are overpossessive or overindulgent, as well as fathers who are too passive, too withdrawn, or too much absent from the home, promote abnormal passivity in boys.

In normal child-parent relationships the identification of the child with the parents results in a child gaining control of his feelings for himself as he fashions himself into an adult of the appropriate sex. However, when there is overcontrol, or no control, a child does not learn how to get control of himself and may react by withdrawing into himself simply because it is safer. He does not learn how to cope with new situations, becomes timid and remains childlike or infantile. The turning-in may be undesirably gratifying because problems are avoided in dealing with other children; fantasies and autoerotic behavior provide substitute satisfaction. He is loath to give up this behavior until he overcomes his inhibitions; only then will he be able to get greater satisfaction from more mature experiences.

Persistent inhibition in pre-school children leads to failure in learning. They are unadventuresome in exploring, and fail to show curiosity about new experiences with things and people. A lack of skill persists because of failure to practice. The child does not permit himself to learn. Children who are struggling with their need to be aggressive and with inhibitions which are self-imposed or set up by others, sometimes end up being well-controlled during the day, but suffer at night from interrupted sleep, nightmares, sleepwalking and so on.

Passivity in a variety of forms is not uncommon in children who are adopted. It is as if they are afraid to show their true selves, lest they lose their new parents. Such behavior may be present for several weeks or months after adoption, but then paradoxically as the child begins to feel more comfortable, this behavior is reversed. The loving and obedient child becomes disobedient, angry and spiteful. This change confuses parents who often find the new traits objectionable. They do not realize that the child is demonstrating good health in the way he is dealing with his new environment and his developmental needs. They tend to view him merely in terms of goodness and badness, whereas he is now so secure that he can risk being disobedient.

As the parent can continue to be accepting and loving despite his "badness," but nevertheless consistent and fair in discipline, the child learns how to deal with his instinctual needs. He finds his place in the new family and is assured of the lasting affection of his new parents. He becomes less "bad" as his testing shows that the security of the family is firmly based. When parents threaten adopted children with punishment, even without saying that they will return them from where they have come, children fear the worst which is abandonment. Anxiety arising from these feelings may lead to an exaggeration of traits parents find obnoxious.

By their play children disclose in fantasy their real struggles with growing up and having relationships with adults and peers. A parent may get clues about such conflicts and feelings by watching and listening to the recurring themes. Such play is self-healing, as well as instructive to the observers.

As parents describe the child's behavior in general and in play specifically the physician can listen attentively and with empathy to their problems, their concerns and their methods of dealing with a child's behavior. He can look for clues in the child's behavior and suggest that the parents also consider what the child is attempting to accomplish by it. In other words, he demonstrates how the parents may gain some insight into the meaning of the child's behavior.

Nursery school may be advised for the shy child to provide experiences which make him more outgoing, more talkative, and more able to demonstrate his emotions. The teachers will have further suggestions for the parents in how to make and keep good relationships with peers.

In families where a father is non-existent or not much involved with the boy, substitutes should be sought. Grandfathers, uncles, recreational leaders and teachers often are competent substitutes for fathers. With the shy child, parents may have to make special efforts at bringing children into the home as playmates. This may be difficult to do when the child lives in a community where there are few or no children of similar age. Parents faced with this recognize the handicap and try to take steps to move to a community where there are children of similar age and interests.

Children who are excessively fearful, withdrawn and clinging, as well as their counterparts who have unmanageable aggressive and antisocial tendencies, are best cared for in residential treatment if ambulatory treatment is not effective. This may be in day hospitals for disturbed children, or in those providing 24 hours per day care. Unfortunately, such facilities both for private and non-paying patients are too rare in this country.

Occasionally nursery schools set up special groups in day care, for long or short term treatment. For example, children who have experienced a death in the family, or a mental illness in a parent, often react with symptoms of grief and depression, or with impulsive acting out. They need emergency care. A nursery school teacher with experience in this, or one who works under the supervision of a psychiatrist may work with 2 or 3 children in a group, for 1 or 2 hours, 1 to 5 times weekly.

By giving special attention to each child, communication is easier and the child may be reached. The child "opens up," reveals his worries, shares them. Often children who cannot work out a problem by discussion can bring it to a satisfactory solution in play fantasies. Painting and story telling have therapeutic value. Stories are selected from folklore in which there are human problems whose solution is told rather graphically by somebody like a hero. Water play, puppetry, building with bricks, are other tools especially when their use is prompted by an astute nursery school teacher. Children and teacher may cook together, prepare lunch and eat a meal. Since feeding difficulties are largely featured in the troubles of the under-5 age group, such lunch making and eating together have special therapeutic value. As he secures understanding, support, encouragement and protection from the teacher he begins to lose some of his shyness, or if over-active quiets down. One sign of improvement is when the child plays according to his own independent fantasy.

Nursery school therapy brings immediate relief to the parents because the separation permits them to live their own lives for a brief period each day. Additional help comes when the parents are given counseling by the physician or by a social worker. Day-hospital treatment, or special nursery school activity is sometimes preferable to individual treatment with a psychiatrist as children with more or less similar problems can contribute a great deal to each other and it is less costly.

Chapter 6

SCHOOL AGE AND PRE-ADOLESCENCE
(5 to 12 years)

SCHOOL AGE AND PRE-ADOLESCENCE

Tasks in Process

CHILD

To master greater physical prowess.

To further establish self identity and sex role.

To work towards greater independence from parents.

To become aware of world-at-large.

To develop peer and other relationships.

To acquire learning, new skills and a sense of industry.

PARENT(S)

To help child's emancipation from parents.

To reinforce self-identification and independence.

To provide positive pattern of social and sex role behavior.

To acclimatize child to world-at-large.

To facilitate learning, reasoning, communication and experiencing.

To promote wholesome moral and ethical values.

Acceptable Behavioral Characteristics

CHILD

General good health, greater body competence, acute sensory perception.

Pride and self confidence; less dependence on parents.

Better impulse control.

Ambivalence re dependency, separation and new experiences.

Accepts own sex role; psychosexual expression in play and fantasy.

Equates parents with peers and other adults.

Aware of natural world (life, death, birth, science); subjective but realistic about world.

Competitive but well organized in play; enjoys peer interaction.

Regard for collective obedience to social laws, rules and fair play.

Explores environment; school and neighborhood basic to social-learning experience.

Cognition advancing; intuitive thinking advancing to concrete operational level; responds to learning.

Speech becomes reasoning and expressive tool; thinking still egocentric.

PARENT(S)

Ambivalent towards child's separation but encourage independence.

Mixed feelings about parent-surrogates but help child to accept them.

Encourage child to participate outside the home.

Set appropriate model of social and ethical behavior and standards.

Take pleasure in child's developing skills and abilities.

Understand and cope with child's behavior.

Find other gratifications in life (activity, employment).

Are supportive towards child as required.

92

(5 to 12 years)

Minimal Psychopathology

CHILD

Anxiety and oversensitivity to new experiences (school, relationships, separation).

Lack of attentiveness; learning difficulties, disinterest in learning.

Acting out: lying, stealing, temper outbursts; inappropriate social behavior.

Regressive behavior (wetting, soiling, crying, fears).

Appearance of compulsive mannerisms (tics, rituals).

Somatic illness: eating and sleeping problems, aches, pains, digestive upsets.

Fear of illness and body injury.

Difficulties and rivalry with peers, siblings, adults; constant fighting.

Destructive tendencies strong; temper tantrums.

Inability or unwillingness to do things for self.

Moodiness and withdrawal; few friends or personal relationships.

PARENT(S)

Disinclination to separate from child; or prematurely hastening separation.

Signs of despondency, apathy, hostility.

Foster fears, dependence, apprehension.

Disinterested in or rejecting of child.

Overly critical and censuring; undermine child's confidence.

Inconsistent in discipline or control; erratic in behavior.

Offer a restrictive, overly moralistic model.

Extreme Psychopathology

CHILD

Extreme withdrawal, apathy, depression, grief, self-destructive tendencies.

Complete failure to learn. Speech difficulty, especially stuttering.

Extreme and uncontrollable anti-social behavior (aggression, destruction, chronic lying, stealing, intentional cruelty to animals).

Severe obsessive-compulsive behavior (phobias, fantasies, rituals).

Inability to distinguish reality from fantasy.

Excessive sexual exhibitionism, eroticism, sexual assaults on others.

Extreme somatic illness: failure to thrive, anorexia, obesity, hypochondriasis, abnormal menses.

Complete absence or deterioration of personal and peer relationships.

PARENT(S)

Extreme depression and withdrawal; rejection of child.

Intense hostility; aggression towards child.

Uncontrollable fears, anxieties, guilts.

Complete inability to function in family role.

Severe moralistic prohibition of child's independent strivings.

Advancing Levels of Maturation

The child of school age and his parents face some problems which are extensions of those met earlier, as well as new ones stemming from experiences in school and in the wider community. The primary tasks faced are those relating to further establishment of his identity and sex role, further separation from parents, a new and closer relationship to his peer group, and the development of a sense of industry in attempts to acquire information, new skills and techniques in learning.

The tasks of the parent relate to those of the child. While the mother continues to have a role which seems to have some primacy, that of the father is equally significant in setting models of adult behavior and sex role, in helping the child to emancipate himself from the close ties with the family and to facilitate learning and new experiences.

The behavioral characteristics of the school child are varied and distinct. He is generally healthy. Medical contacts and hospitalization are infrequent, so there is less reason for concern about body function and health. Except for numerous minor respiratory infections and the common communicable diseases, complaints about illness ("feeling sick," "having pain") are apt to be related more to events which upset the child and parents psychologically. School attendance is the most prominent of these.

When the school child is physically sick or has a physical disability like deafness or poor eyesight, he is better able to comprehend the reasons for his defects and discomforts, and the purposes of the treatment. He can ask questions and be given information which make situations more comprehensible and therefore less frightening. He is better able to tolerate separation from family. This is not to deny that he still is capable of being anxious and that his care must embrace psychologic as well as physical measures.

In his physical development the child shows greater skill in motor performance and coordination. His greater physical prowess invites more risk taking and this accounts for some accidents. The number of children having accidents remains high and some are particularly prone to injury. This is the time to stress safety and teach the child to follow rules preparatory to the time when family and teacher supervision is not possible, and when accident prevention depends on early training and conditioning. The role of the physician is to help parents, children and school personnel plan play activities which permit children to explore their environment and test their abilities without undue risk to themselves or to others. Lessons in automobile construction and driving should begin in class rooms in the later part of this age period.

In this phase of development the child accepts his sex role and enjoys emphasizing it in play with his peers. He is tolerant of the opposite sex but participates infrequently and rather unwillingly in their activities. The school age period is referred to as the latency period in psychoanalytic terms, in the sense of one with less evidence of direct sexual and aggressive impulse activity and sexual conflict. In reality this appears to be a matter of relativity.

Some children display greater amounts of interest and concern about sex, and frequently engage in solitary and interpersonal sexual activities. These may be evidence of arrests in development or acts precipitated by stimulation of others. Also they may come from upsetting experiences such as failing to learn in school, faulty peer-group relationships, anxiety about health, or grief and mourning.

Parents also vary in the amount of concern they have about their children's sex behavior. Some are permissive of masturbation, others go out of their way to check up whenever a child enters the bathroom, are suspicious that he is preoccupied with sex thoughts and begin to see danger when there is no cause. In other children, sex play is less overt and the parents are reassured by its seeming absence.

It is certain that school children do think and fantasy about sexual and aggressive impulses and conflicts. Where these items are under excessive or ineffectual modification, repression extends into other areas of behavior, particularly school learning. Sex activities most often include autoerotic activity, mutual masturbation and exhibitionism, especially among boys when they compare size of penis and force of urinary stream. Such behavior must be viewed as experimental learning about oneself. It is not pathologic in itself.

Both sexes may attempt to look at and examine the other, particularly the genitals of children younger than themselves. This rarely goes to a point of sex play or attempts at intercourse. Children are overstimulated by parents who exhibit themselves, who talk excessively about sex behavior, and who are preoccupied with sex instruction.

The school aged child's play is better organized, often imaginative and ingenious. There is regard for rules and fair play with better impulse control. He is aware of the need for collective obedience to rules and of the advantages of group membership. Leadership qualities are often demonstrated clearly in this age, and it may be predicted that when present they will remain throughout childhood into adult life.

Parents are equated more with peers and other adults although they continue to hold positions of importance. The child still uses them as models of behavior and is dependent on them. But as the school and neighborhood become more important vehicles for experiencing and learning the child begins to question the all-knowingness of parents and to experience conflicts of loyalty.

Sometimes parents bring questions to a physician about a child's moral and ethical behavior, especially lying, stealing and cheating. Moral values for the young child are generalized as they are learned. He views moral laws as absolute values in real things. Moral values and rules exist as an indivisible part of the object. For example, the command "do not touch the ink" becomes the property of the ink. Ink is something not to be touched. Father and obedience to father are viewed as one. Disobedience is an infringement of adult authority rather than a violation of a moral obligation. Naughty words are bad because they break adult-imposed taboos. Reproof and punishment are expected as natural consequences of misbehavior. Guilt makes him seek atonement.

He achieves this by obsessive-compulsive behavior, by rituals and other means of self-punishment. A child of this kind may develop his own taboos about thoughts and acts, with compulsions such as when he does not permit himself to touch certain objects or persons, or even to look at them. He imputes magic power to thoughts and feelings. He avoids cripples to prevent harm to himself or others. The childish game of never stepping on cracks in a sidewalk, lest they "break your mother's back," has the element of self-punishment and magical protection. It is more than a simple rhyming game. This is what Piaget calls a child's employment of "imminent justice," whereby he brings a verdict of guilty and subsequently inflicts punishment upon himself whenever he commits what he or someone else considers a wrong.

Children conform to adult rules because of respect and constraint towards adult authority and prestige, yet they are confused by rules which adults have for themselves which seem elastic and not absolute.

Sometimes children cheat and steal, despite their parents' prohibition, because they have witnessed such acts in their parents. In play and fantasy, the school-aged child uses the rules and values of his elders. Parents are sometimes surprised when they see themselves "played back" as unfair, dishonest and unfaithful. In school a child learns how to turn for guidance to multiple authorities rather than to parents alone. He also looks to his peers. This influence can be good, or it can be misleading as when group cheating is engaged in because "everybody does it." Occasionally children steal as a one-time experiment in defying the authorities or in order to win the attention and respect of peers. Such prowess gains greater respect than success in school, not only from peers but even from some parents.

A young child does not consider the multiple motives or consequences of his act; a lie is judged by the degree of disobedience involved. He does not see the implications of deceit but only that it is an act which he has considered for an immediate gain.

In cognitive terms, the "conscience finds its anchoring points in newly acquired centers of mutual respect and awareness of collective obedience." The sense of morality is internalized as the child incorporates the values, standards and expectations of his elders. A lack of such guidance interferes with moral and ethical development.

A clinical problem of this etiology is the delinquent child. The habitual liar, the chronic thief, the child who acts out impulsively without regard for the welfare of others often has lacked opportunity to imitate and identify with parents who might have helped him deal with issues in more acceptable ways. The methods and techniques used might be appropriate for what the child is attempting to gain for himself, but by society's standards they are inappropriate. Some of these children have reached a point where they are no longer able to distinguish reality from fantasy. This is a severe psychopathologic reaction which may represent a character neurosis or a beginning psychosis.

Sometimes stealing, so-called, comes about not because a child cannot distinguish between what is his and what belongs to others, but rather because his place in the family is so undifferentiated from others that he does not distinguish himself as separate. He takes things as if they were his; everything that belongs to the family is viewed as possessed equally by all its members. As a school child approaches adolescence, he will make a strong demand to have his own property separated from that of others, but he may still be inclined to take without permission property which belongs to his parents. Rifling the mother's pocketbook at will without telling the mother is viewed by her as stealing. When faced with the so-called theft, the child denies that he has done wrong and explains that he has merely taken what he believed was his, or has "borrowed."

The school-aged child is more aware than the pre-schooler about the facts of life, birth and death. Now he not only questions his origin biologically, but is interested in the process of birth, and increasingly the acts of procreation. He tends not to pursue these questions because he senses that they are taboo for many parents and they do not feel at ease in giving explanations.

Although talking about birth and sexual intercourse is difficult for some parents, it is even harder to explain death. Children want to know, as does everyone else, why people die and what happens after death. Parents must answer these questions honestly and as best they can in keeping with their own beliefs. Children grieve the death of parents and other relatives, and of pets. In addition to the feeling of loss and sorrow, there may be guilt. Even children of this age, who comprehend more, tend to accuse themselves to some degree for the death of loved ones. Prolonged grief constitutes mental depression. Psychotic episodes of a manic-depressive variety are rarely encountered in the school-age child but periods of discouragement and depression are not rare. There is a marked rise in frequency of suicides in childhood in the second decade of life. (See Suicide, pages 217–222.)

The child who adapts best is the one who developed trust in parents in the earlier years and whose parents have become trusting of him. When problems arise, the pediatrician serves well when he helps parents see their conflicts and those of the child. He should guide them in ways of gradually allowing the child to participate with them and with others outside the home and to accept instruction from substitute adults about crucial aspects of human experience in the adult world.

Mothers need to find new sources of gratification, sometimes in service to other children, sometimes in employment outside the home, to compensate for the reduced mothering of their own child. The mother who cannot adjust may be confronted with old problems. She may become depressed and require psychiatric help. The pediatrician will notice the symptoms of this from the ways she handles her child, is unable to cope, and by signs of dejection and apathy. If the mother's behavior indicates, with her permission it may be best to talk with her husband and share concern with him. Another approach is to interview husband and wife together in the hope that either one will raise questions about what is to be done in regard to their emotional reactions to the child's behavior.

School Learning Problems

The anxiety of starting school is to be expected from most children. It may be less for those who have already experienced such separation when going to nursery school and who have learned that it is only temporary. However, nursery school is no sure preventive against the development of school anxiety and phobias. Children who separated with difficulty when introduced to nursery school (or whose parents experienced such anxiety) should be marked by the pediatrician. They may be prone to show fearfulness in all new school situations. The anxiety may appear overtly as extensive and irrational fear and phobias, or as temper tantrums, complaints about body pain (especially "stomachache"), nightmares, enuresis, loss of appetite, and others. There may be a carry over into school learning as when the child fails to learn, or even to attempt to learn.

Normally the sense organs are highly developed so that perception is acute and this facilitates school learning. Where there are problems of learning, assessment of the physical health and especially of vision and hearing ability is a primary responsibility of the physician. When teachers and parents complain of a child's lack of attention, this may be due to failure to comprehend on a physical, emotional or intellectual basis. There should be concern also regarding physical growth and nutrition, particularly thinness and obesity.

The management of these problems entails a thorough physical examination, occasionally laboratory testing, medical treatment if necessary, and invariably psychologic helping. (See Psychosomatic Disorders, page 110.) Conflicts in the child about eating certain foods may have persisted from early childhood, along with clashes with parents about food and eating habits. When this is associated with learning or behavior difficulties the problems are usually so deep-seated that psychiatric treatment is indicated. Enuresis is uncommon. Although constipation is frequent, it is less often complained about; fecal soiling and encopresis are rare.

The school child has pride in himself and in his accomplishments. He is competitive and gains self-confidence with each success in peer play and in school achievement. At first, however, he has mixed feelings about leaving home to attend school. He finds it difficult to deal with new loyalties to peers and adults. He may (like the adolescent) try to find reasons why he should leave the parents. One unconscious technique is to fantasy the parents as unloving and fault finding, as persons who are desirous of getting rid of the child. He responds with hostility, as if he were retaliating against their hostility. This is a "normal" paranoia, and provides justification for the child and the adolescent to function well away from home without regret and with less guilt.

It is the task of the parents to accept such behavior with equanimity and to help him more or less subtly to find parent surrogates who are competent and responsible people. To fight hostility with rejection may set off even more unpleasant behavior, some of which may take the form of regression, as in greater dependence and unwillingness to leave the home and mother for any reason.

Most parents accept the greater independence of the child and encourage it. Mothers often have some feelings of apprehension and even of loss when the child goes off to school. Will he be able to cope with the schooling, with the group activities and with the strange teachers? Some resent the influence of teachers whom they view ambivalently. They are expected to teach but not to act as parent surrogates. They may be viewed as rivals, although often the parents' apprehension is their vicarious way of experiencing their own days as students.

Such mothers abet a child's disinclination to separate, and it is their holding back more than his fear or phobia that produces early school problems. At the other extreme are those parents who push their child into boarding schools and are overtly rejecting.

According to Piaget, the time of beginning elementary school (5 to 7 years) is marked as the phase of intuitive thought. But like the earlier period of life, this is still a time of pre-operational thought. There is widening of social interest in the world-at-large, less egocentricity and more social participation. The child is less passively accepting of the environment as he experiences it and more able to react to it realistically.

8

Thinking and reasoning are acted out. The child tries to coordinate his subjective versions of the world with the real world around him. During this phase he increasingly acts in a consistent pattern of reasoning. Piaget says he behaves "as if he intuitively knew what life was about, and this marks the real beginnings of cognition."

The child begins to use words and thoughts as trial actions. Much as he formerly used his motor apparatus to act out his thinking, now he begins to employ speech to express thinking. His perceptions are still colored by his personal preconceptions, and his thinking is still egocentric to a great degree. This means that his views may be at variance with those of his elders and with the real world. He usually gives evidence of thinking of only one idea at a time. Thinking in terms of the whole is not characteristic.

By a variety of processes, with benefit of maturation and the help of parents, teachers and peers, the young school child develops from the phase of intuitive thinking to that of concrete operations and finally that of formal operations. The details of this development and the theories explaining them are best studied in texts by Piaget and his interpreters.

For our purpose it is enough to point out that when all goes well, the physician is not consulted about children's learning. But failure to learn in school is probably the most important reason for children being admitted to child guidance clinics today, and most of them are referred by non-psychiatric physicians.

School learning problems therefore stem from a variety of causes: acute and chronic ill health, central and peripheral nervous system disease, intrapsychic and interpersonal factors. Often there are combinations of noxious conditions, as when disorganization of brain function interferes with a child's interpersonal environment and/or emotional factors assume a dominant influence.

The following case histories describe the pernicious psychologic influences on school learning due to intra family disturbance and/or physical disability.

Case of Fred S., age 11 years: School Failure; A reactive psychogenic disturbance

Presenting Complaint. Failing in school for past 6 months. Previous academic record excellent. Distractible in class, cannot concentrate, does not do homework, writing has become poor and there are times when boy seems withdrawn and lost in daydreams.

History. Infancy and early childhood normal. Born at term, birthweight 7½ pounds. Mother's pregnancy uneventful. Infancy uncomplicated and no problems of eating or sleeping. Received regular pediatric check-ups and mother took advice willingly. She had never seemed apprehensive, overprotective or overpermissive. She was considered an "ideal mother."

Attended nursery school from 3 to 5 years of age, accommodated well, and had no trouble separating from mother. At 4 years of age he developed pneumonia and was hospitalized for 2 weeks. Toilet training which had been successful regressed, much to the chagrin of the mother. Boy resented new training attempts, developed blinking tics of eyes which lasted about 2 months. Tics disappeared when toilet training was again accomplished. Boy continued to talk about hospital and feared return. He made parents promise that he would not be taken to hospital again.

He started kindergarten at 5½ years with some apprehension about leaving mother for the first week but then settled in. He had some of the common communicable diseases, without complication, after starting school. Enjoyed kindergarten, was active in group play, showed good motor coordination and enjoyed music rhythm. Learned to copy numbers and letters in first grade, and was reading well at third grade. He was promoted each year so that now at age 11 he was in the sixth grade.

Teachers became puzzled about this boy's change in learning ability and school performance. Always considered an excellent student, friendly, compliant, and energetic, for the past 6 months he had a "changed personality." Homework was either not done or brought in unfinished and inaccurate. School examinations were failed and often uncompleted. He seemed to resent being reminded of his excellent record. The teacher found him hard to reach. Peers considered him angry, uncooperative, and secretive.

The father had reacted to school report with anger, reduction of allowance and threats not to send him to college. Father complained that college admission to the school of his choice would be difficult because of academic failures. Boy was angry with father and both were in frequent conflict verbally. At one time father had hit the boy. Mother pleaded with child to try hard, to concentrate, to think of his future, to obey his father. Neither parent had talked about their own incompatibility to the patient.

Family. Father, 41, junior executive in an advertising agency. Ivy League graduate, hoped his son would follow his pattern educationally and vocationally. No financial troubles until the past 6 months when he fell in love with his secretary, talked of divorce, began to drink excessively and found that his income could not meet expenses. Mother, 38, healthy, a housewife who enjoyed her life at home and with the children, was shocked when approached by her husband about divorce and had reacted to this with negativism and appeals to him for reconciliation. These had failed. Patient had heard mother and father argue, but they felt he did not know the basis of their marital problems. Their two younger female children recently had presented problems of bedwetting and night terrors.

Examination. Patient was well-nourished and well-developed, obviously not sick. He was unwilling to talk, seemed despondent, and when asked about his plans broke into tears. He refused to confide in pediatrician about difficulties. He was told his physical examination was negative but that he seemed worried and the physician would like to talk with him again if he was willing. It was agreed that the boy would call for his own appointment. Mother accepted this recommendation.

Three weeks later, after boy had refused to go to school for a week, and expulsion was threatened, boy asked for an interview. He now confided his feelings to the pediatrician, talked in length about his knowledge of the parents' quarrels and their threat to leave each other. He still loved his parents, even his father, but was puzzled by their behavior and felt that he was being rejected as a stranger. Boy raised the question about going to boarding school where he could avoid hearing the parents' quarrels and where he could get a new start academically. He agreed that the physician should talk with both parents and inform them of his concerns and his desires.

Both parents were interviewed 2 days later, were surprised that their son was so insightful about their behavior and said they would consider boarding school placement. It was suggested that they seek marital counselling. They accepted referral to the University Department of Psychiatry for that purpose. Seen there for 6 months at weekly intervals, parents became reconciliated, but since boy still pressed for boarding school this was arranged. In the last months of the academic year, boy's performance improved but never attained that achieved before.

Two years later, the boy had graduated from boarding school with honors and returned to his community to enter public high school. The reconciliation of the parents had worked out satisfactorily in the opinion of both parents.

Case of Ruth Jane, age 12 years: Acute School Avoidance; Family stress

Presenting Complaint. Referred by her pediatrician to the pediatric out-patient department because of refusal to go to school. She had been out of school 4 weeks. The onset was at the time of her second menstrual period in January, when she stayed at home

Thursday and Friday because of cramps. She felt better over the weekend, but on Monday developed vomiting and diarrhea. This was diagnosed as virus gastroenteritis, and she was advised to stay home all week.

The following Monday she started to school, but fell out the door, spraining her wrist. She went on to school at her mother's insistence, but began to have vomiting and diarrhea again. She was sent home by the school physician, and her pediatrician recommended that she stay home for the rest of the week. The following week she had constipation and vague abdominal pain, for which she continued to remain at home. By this time it became apparent that it was difficult for her to return to school, and referral to clinic was arranged to evaluate the physical and psychologic factors which might be responsible.

Ruth Jane was an honor student at a parochial school. She was president of her class until she had been out of school 2 weeks; then this office was taken from her. She wanted to go to the public junior high school after this school year, but expected to finish the year in parochial school. Although she had a strict teacher, there had been no known upsetting events in school at the time Ruth Jane stopped attending.

She usually missed about 10 to 14 days from school each year. At the age of 10, when she had her tonsils removed, she did not return for 6 weeks. The month before that illness she had stayed at home 3 days for "grippe" and again 1 week at the time of the maternal grandmother's death.

Family. The parents were in their early fifties. The father was a roller grinder. The only sibling was a 10-year-old sister, who was in fifth grade and had no school problems. The family owned their home and Ruth Jane had her own room.

The mother talked briefly with a social worker on this first visit and revealed that the father was alcoholic, had liver disease, and was "killing himself" with drink. When he would come home nearly comatose, the mother would berate him severely in front of the children. She was on the verge of a separation.

Examination. Ruth Jane was a tall, well-nourished, healthy-appearing adolescent girl. She was quiet, reserved, polite, self-contained and intelligent. She resented the implication that there were any emotional problems keeping her from returning to school. Physical examination showed no abnormality. The initial impression was "virus gastroenteritis but rule out school phobia."

Ruth Jane was reassured about her good health and encouraged to return to school. Next day she complained of a sudden sore throat on the way to school and refused to go. Her mother became angry and threatened to drag her. When the patient screamed, the mother took her home and sent her to her room to "lie and rot." The next 2 days Ruth Jane continued to complain of sore throat and made no attempt to go to school.

The clinic physician, a senior medical student, telephoned each day, talking with both mother and daughter. He suggested that the mother diminish her punitive approach, let Mary Jane out of bed, and try to help her gently but firmly to get to school. He helped Ruth Jane set a date for her return on the last day of the week. On this day her mother drove her to school. She complained of mucus in her throat and vomited shortly after arrival. She was helped to stay, and was welcomed by both her teacher and her classmates. She was pleasantly surprised that the day was not hard.

Next week was a midwinter vacation from school. She worked hard at making up lessons she had missed, in expectation of returning to school the next Monday. On her second clinic visit, during this week, she expressed confidence in continuing in school. Although she had been afraid on the day she went, she had pride in her ability to go anyway. Her fear was expressed as fear of further digestive symptoms. She brushed aside any efforts to help her talk about her home situation. She expressed happiness in having returned to school and did not anticipate further trouble.

The social worker talked with the mother again on this occasion. The mother described herself as nervous, volatile, frequently explosive. There were long-standing marital problems, including marked disagreements about the care of the children. The mother had talked with the priest about separation. The father accused the mother of being dominated by her sister, who spoiled the children. The mother had felt keenly the deaths of her mother and her mother-in-law in the past 3 months.

The father looked yellow and sickly, at least 15 years older than his age, which worried Ruth Jane who asked the mother not to tell anyone of her father's condition. The mother replied that she felt it was important to discuss it with the social worker. She gave permission for the doctor to discuss the family strife with Ruth Jane.

The mother described the preparation of her daughter for menarche, trying to present it as a normal function, but with many prohibitions and possibly with frightening anticipation of discomfort. The mother talked freely and seemed to gain some comfort in sharing her burdens with the social worker. She seemed to realize that the marital stress might be related to Ruth Jane's problem in going to school.

It was planned that the girl return to clinic in 2 weeks to discuss her feelings about full-time return to school, to have an opportunity to ask questions about her development and her menstrual periods, and if she wished, to talk over the impact of the family situation on her. This appointment was cancelled by the mother because Ruth Jane was attending school, and no need was felt for another visit. The physician talked by telephone with the patient who expressed happiness in the school situation. An invitation was extended to her and the mother to return to clinic if they felt it would be helpful sometime in the future. A report was sent back to the referring physician, who may be in a better position than the clinic doctor to go on helping this young girl with her concerns about her family and growing up.

Impressions. This was a 12-year-old girl, who had been out of school for 4 weeks with complaints of gastrointestinal symptoms, sore throat and sprained wrist. Other contributing causes may have been the deaths of two grandmothers within 3 months, hepatic disease and alcoholism in the father, severe marital discord between the parents with threats of separation, fears about menarche and adolescent development, and desire to change from parochial to regular school.

By means of two clinic visits and several telephone calls, a pediatrician (senior medical student) was able to reassure himself about her physical health and with confidence so advise her. He was also able to help her understand a little of the relationship of feelings to somatic symptoms, and support that part of her which wished to return to school and resume her place with her peers. The encouragement, even the insistence, to return to school probably prevented the development of what often is called a "school phobia." The longer a child stays out of school, the harder it is for him to return. If not actually having a phobia, such a child certainly is apprehensive in most instances about leaving home.

Case of Dennis T., age 10 years: Poor School Record; Deafness and emotional stress

Presenting Complaint. For the past several years Dennis exhibited "funny behavior"—headshaking, grimacing, and kicking heels together when walking. He had become sullen and showed temper tantrums at home when chided about his poor school record. Although none of these traits were ever absent, each varied in intensity from time to time. Sleep was quiet and restful; excitement seemed to precipitate the facial movements.

The school teacher and school nurse notified parents about their concern because the facial movements interfered with his concentration when studying and disturbed his classmates. Mother ac-

knowledged awareness of her son's behavior, had scolded and
ridiculed him, but this had been without influence. Father, who
wore a hearing aid, paid no attention to the patient, being withdrawn and inattentive. Mother sought pediatric help when school
threatened to keep Dennis in fourth grade for second year.

History. This was uneventful in terms of health and development.
Boy averaged five or six colds a year, frequently complicated with
earache. Tonsillectomy had been suggested several times because
of otitis media and enlargement of tonsils.

Family. Father, aged 45, was a laborer, had recurrent ear trouble
as a child leading to loss of hearing bilaterally. He was sensitive
about his deafness, took little part in rearing children. Earnings
barely sustained the family. Mother was 38, a healthy housewife
who worried about her own health but sought no medical help. She
was concerned also about her three children. The oldest son was
12 years and had rheumatic fever twice; a 9-year-old daughter was
underdeveloped, anemic and a slow learner.

Examination. Dennis was in the tenth percentile in height and
weight for his age. He was tense, jumpy but cooperative. He
comprehended directions but spoke little. There were grimaces of
the mouth, eyeblinking and shaking of the head, all exacerbated
when blood was drawn for hematologic studies.

He said that he could not control his head and face movements
and that they relieved his "nervousness." His speech was somewhat
infantile and monotonal. Dennis said that he was worried about
school and attributed his difficulties to not being able to comprehend
the "hard work" in the classroom. He seemed to have trouble
understanding the questions of the physician, but this improved as
the interrogator's voice became louder.

Physical examination revealed nothing to suggest central nervous
system or brain damage. Tonsils were large; a watch was heard
only when held next to each ear. Psychologic testing gave the following results: By Wechsler Intelligence Scale (Verbal) I.Q. 77,
(Performance) I.Q. 118. In the examination he was tense, anxious,
angry and testing was done with difficulty because of his seeming
inattentiveness.

Impressions. The boy's school learning problem as well as his
behavior at home were believed to be related to his deafness and
to his emotional state. The former was considered to be caused by
physical pathologic conditions (enlarged tonsils and adenoids and
infection). The tics and the complex of anxiety, tension and anger
were probably reactions to his inability to function well in school
and to the manner in which his parents dealt with him. Although
the father reacted to his own deafness by withdrawing, the boy

was responding to this attitude and to the pressure put upon him by mother and teacher by becoming anxious and angry.

Removal of the tonsils and adenoids was recommended and carried out. Four months later when the hearing was unimproved and audiometry showed bilateral deafness, a hearing aid was prescribed. The mother was calmer about her child's tics, especially when his school teacher reported an improvement in his attitude towards learning and his achievement. Remedial teaching was provided to help Dennis make up the lag in his school work. The father continued to be absorbed with his own problems and continued to pay little direct attention to his children.

Two years later the tics had disappeared with the exception of occasional eye-blinking when reading aloud. Ophthalmologic examination showed no disease. It was believed that there was still some tension around learning and in his relationships with parents and peers. He was considered an average student at this time.

Brain Damage (Chronic Brain Syndromes)

These disorders result from "relatively permanent, more or less irreversible, diffuse impairment of cerebral tissue function." Such impairment may occur from congenital cranial anomalies, prenatal and perinatal brain injury, infection of the central nervous system, brain trauma, convulsive disorders, disturbances of metabolism, growth and nutrition, neoplasms and heredodegenerative diseases.

There are no specific types of personality disorders associated with these brain syndromes. The differing symptoms depend on the difference in the pathologic condition as well as on the nature of the child's normal, constitutional potentials and the psychologic factors in child and parents. Some children are better endowed than others despite what appears to be a similiar amount of the same pathologic condition.

The way a child and his parents perceive his limitations also differs. Greater insight, more optimistic personalities, better economic circumstances and excellent professional guidance combine to facilitate rehabilitation. Any combination of these assets is beneficial.

There is a core of symptoms which is central to most brain syndromes; hyperactivity, distractibility and impulsivity, disorders in perceptual motor functions, difficulty in spatial orientation and in cerebral integration and organizational capacities. Reading, writing and abstract concept formation are faulty. Concepts of time and space are difficult to comprehend. There is also extreme emotional lability, a short attention span, social incompetence, vacillating work habits in school and meddlesomeness. These traits are also found in some autistic children, giving rise to the belief that their difficulties are due to brain damage. The term central nervous system dysfunction may be a more accurate description of what can be diagnosed. (See Autism, pages 211–213.)

The diagnosis of organicity should be made on the evidence of brain damage and on the presence of the constellation of symptoms just mentioned. Specific neurologic signs are not always demonstrable or are elicited only by experts in developmental and neurologic examination. When present, they usually consist of abnormal extension of the arms when the eyes are closed, choreiform or mild choreo-athetoid movements, awkwardness in movements and in walking on a line, difficulty in skipping and standing on one foot. Writing and picture drawing show synkinesia. The electroencephalogram may be normal, or show diffuse abnormalities. Unfortunately, an electroencephalogram is often interpreted differently by different experts.

The diagnosis of brain damage, sometimes with the prefix "minimal," is often made when there is no history of brain damage and when there are no abnormal neurologic signs. Since there is no verified etiology, this is a misnomer. The diagnosis is misleading and detrimental in that it frequently stigmatizes children who are then treated as if they were incapable of learning the usual tasks of education, and seem unworthy of the efforts of educators.

Until several years ago, the diagnosis of minimal brain damage when applied to infants and pre-school children prevented them from being adopted. When it was realized that most of them developed normally ultimately, without neurologic residue, adoption practices were changed permitting earlier adoption. It is our impression that the diagnosis of minimal brain damage based primarily on behavioral manifestations has questionable merit, and that even the designation "brain damaged," made only on behavior, must be made with caution because it may lead to inappropriate management.

Many children with brain syndromes are not significantly retarded in intellectual development and have a favorable prognosis if appropriately treated. However, they may show specific learning difficulties, and may function at a mentally retarded level, with psychologic and social factors playing a contributory role. If mental retardation is present, this can be detected through psychologic testing by a competent clinical psychologist.

The brain damaged child can be happy, friendly and outgoing, yet he is viewed by peers and adults as strange and different. Often he is frustrating to teachers and parents. Hence treatment must include the encouragement and support of those persons responsible to educate and rear him.

The role of the pediatrician is that of a member of the diagnostic team, including also a neurologist, psychologist, teacher and a psychiatrist. His task is to convene the services of the others and interpret their findings to the parents and to those colleagues, like the teacher, who could benefit. The pediatric management should also include supervision of medications. (See Medication, pages 199–201.)

Counseling of parents before, during and after psychiatric treatment, is an important function of the non-psychiatric physician or his associates, the social worker and psychologist. The teacher will be responsible for providing the specialized educational resources required.

Case of William C., age 9 years: A brain-damaged boy

Presenting complaint. Restless and slow in school; cannot concentrate; does not follow instructions; excessive daydreaming; temper tantrums. He had trouble adjusting to kindergarten because he was impulsive, could not sit still and his play was disorganized. Nevertheless he was promoted to the first grade where he continued to show the behavior just described. He found it difficult to use a pencil or crayon and could not even copy circles and squares.

He repeated first grade where he seemed to relate better to children but continued to make comments which seemed irrelevant, did not learn to copy numbers and had no interest in reading. At 7 years of age in a group intelligence test he scored an I.Q. of 90. At 9 years, an I.Q. on Stanford-Binet was 86. The psychologist found it difficult to hold his attention, he was easily distracted, became angry when urged to perform. The Bender-Gestalt test was interpreted as showing central nervous system deviation.

History. Mother showed spotting during third month of pregnancy. Born somewhat prematurely, birth weight was 5 pounds. He gained weight slowly in hospital incubator where he remained for 14 days. Feeding and training were difficult because he was slow to learn. He still wets the bed occasionally.

Family. Mother age 44, healthy, but worried over son whom she feels has never been normal like his 3-year-older sister who never presented any problem. Mother wonders whether boy is mentally deficient. Works with him on homework but both her patience and his are soon exhausted and the child becomes angry. Father aged 46, healthy, employed as a chemist and has high educational expectations for both his children.

Examination. Boy was well-nourished, stocky, apprehensive, could not sit still, became surly when asked to remove his clothing. He had trouble unbuttoning his shirt and later was unable to tie shoelaces. With arms extended, slight choreo-athetoid movements of the body, arms and fingers were demonstrated. Electroencephalogram read as showing diffuse abnormalities not consistent with any known lesion.

Impressions. From history and examination, diagnosis of brain dysfunction was made.

Disposition. Boy was placed in a special class which had a few pupils and a teacher trained to deal with the perceptually handicapped. Dexedrine was prescribed. Mother was told to stop working with him on homework. Both parents were advised that child may not have the educational potential that they look for. After 6 months, teacher reported an increased attention span, an interest in reading with greater facility in copying figures and writing numbers.

Psychosomatic Disorders

Bodily disturbances in which emotional factors play a predominant or precipitating role are not limited to any age or phase of development. However, psychosomatic disorders are frequent in school age children. Next to acute respiratory illnesses they are the commonest cause for repeated absence from school.

The child at that age develops illnesses which in natural history and symptomatology resemble more closely those of adults than did the ills of infancy and the pre-school period. For example, ulcerative colitis appears more frequently among school children than among younger individuals, and resembles the adult form, while diarrhea and other gastrointestinal disturbances which appear in infancy do not become colitis in the sense of that associated with older persons.

The mechanisms responsible for the development of psychosomatic disorders are not easily delineated, nor are those factors which are responsible for the illness of some children at certain periods of their lives. The fact that school children react differently to anxiety than do infants, for example, may be because the nervous system is more mature, or because their physiologic responsiveness is based on other intrinsic factors. Also, the school aged child is capable of symbolizing his conflicts and the compromises that the physical and social sides of himself must reach in his development. Just as he is capable of using symbolic communication for learning and understanding in this age period so he may express a conflict symbolically or psychosomatically, with tension expressed as psychologic and physiologic parts of the whole. Human beings react with some degree of similarity to the same stimulus although with great individual difference. This is probably dependent on such things as the constitution, the psychologic vulnerability of that individual at that particular time of his life, and the nature of the general environment or ecology in which the patient is living.

There is merit in considering certain diseases as *psychosomatic* in that the physician is impelled to deal with the psychologic as well as the somatic aspects diagnostically and therapeutically. However, every physician is mindful of the fact there is always an interplay between bodily and emotional states in every illness, and that both psychologic and somatic systems must be considered in dealing with the patient. Hence the terms *comprehensive medicine* or *holistic medical care* are frequently used to designate the ideal management of sick persons; the implication being that treatment of the disease will include psychologic and environmental intervention as well as bodily needs.

Whatever its cause a psychosomatic disorder provokes additional anxiety which may lead to further bodily disturbances and to persistence of the disorder. Asthma is such an illness, in which the symptom leads to its own perpetuation. The patient with respiratory distress becomes anxious. The anxiety in turn further increases the respiratory difficulty, which in turn produces even more apprehension.

In the school age period, as well as in adolescence and the adult years, there is a broad spectrum of illnesses in which there is a sequential relationship between primary emotional stress and bodily disorder. In these it is found that modifying the emotional state leads to relief of symptoms. The spectrum runs from such seemingly innocuous (yet infantile regressive) states such as thumbsucking and fecal soiling, to complicated disorders like ulcerative colitis and the allergies. The commonest disorders in the school age period are those characterized somatically by bodily pain, (particularly headaches and "stomachaches"), anorexia, overeating and obesity, diarrhea, chronic fatigue and allergic disorders. Unexplained fever, presumed to be psychogenic, is not infrequent.

Ulcerative colitis is frequently labeled a psychosomatic disorder and ascribed to faulty parental attitudes in bowel training, with the resultant accumulation of repressed anger and hostility. It is also labeled a somatopsychic disorder with the causes primarily infection, allergy or auto-immunization. The physician generally is consulted about the somatic problems but often he realizes that psychologic components are also more or less involved and require management.

Whatever its origins, ulcerative colitis must be treated as a disease afflicting the *whole person*. His anxiety, overdependence, disturbed family relationships and whatever other psychosocial elements are involved must be treated quite as much as his diarrhea, nutritional deficiency and other physical aberrations.

In general, the mechanisms for the development of a psychosomatic disorder appear to be as follows. The person's constitution, which is itself the result of heredity and life experiences, predisposes an individual to react in certain ways in a stressful or difficult situation. Whether the stress of the new situation is organic or psychologic, the responses will include psychologic and physical reactions. The same situation may not be especially stimulating or anxiety-provoking to others, and the situation may not always be so stressful to this particular patient. However, for some reason or another at the time of the development of the illness, the psychologic stress does have particular meaning as a threat. The person tries to cope, and may succeed partially or not at all. He may have symptoms or he may not.

If the stimulus is repeated or increased in severity, or if the environment becomes more stressful, the residue from the previous reaction may predispose the patient to greater failure of adaptation. Signs and symptoms of somatic illness now appear. The reasons for involvement of a specific organ system are unclear. It is assumed that the choice is unconscious, and that the site is predisposed by either constitutional weakness or a previous trauma. From now on, such a patient will have a predilection for the development of a similar pathologic condition at other times of stress. There is an analogy to the patient who is more prone to develop greater disorder of the heart once he has developed some cardiac condition, however mild it may have been at first.

The prognosis of a psychosomatic disorder may never be made with certainty. Some children recover from the illness and have no recurrence, others have identical and magnified recurrences, while some develop other illnesses as substitutes. In other words, some individuals learn from the first experience how to cope and adapt to stressful situations, even after a severe psychosomatic disorder.

Others seem to cope well, and the symptoms are dormant, while the anxiety is repressed. The disorders are "sleepers," in that there may be a hiatus of several years without recurrence, but one day when circumstances seem appropriate they reappear and may now even become chronic.

The rate of "cure" following attempts at intervention are as unclear as that where cases are not treated at all. Little is known about the natural history and prognosis of psychosomatic conditions. In general, therefore, one must be guarded in predicting the outcome of psychogenic disorders. Nevertheless, every attempt should be made to help children utilize mechanisms which are presumed helpful in coping, in the hope that such efforts will relieve and prevent illness.

In the management of psychosomatic disorders, one must deal not only with the individual who is suffering from the disorder but with his parents. Often the disorders begin with a period of crisis in the life of the child, and the physician must try to determine the nature of the crisis. This is done by careful interviewing of patient, parents and sometimes others like school teachers. A change in the environment of school and home may remove much of the crisis stress. This is all that is required in some cases.

Sometimes a child's symptomatology follows a family pattern as when the school child complains of abdominal pain whenever facing stress. This may be similar to the pattern of the mother who chronically complains of abdominal pain whether related to menstruation, quarrels with husband, or other stress within the family. Children assume and repeat or simulate symptoms of parents, mostly by unconscious identification. Parents may predispose children to anxiety around certain experiences in the manner by which they warn children about the dangers of going to school, crossing streets, taking an airplane ride or whatever new experience. This is not to deny that there may be risk in a situation, but the condition is an expression of the parents' manner and reactions, and in due time the child's reaction.

Therapy for psychosomatic disorders thus includes sustained and adequate physiologic and symptomatic treatment, manipulation and changing of the environment, attempts at modifying parental and family patterns of reacting to stress, and finally in dealing directly with the child's and parents' feelings and attitudes. This may require psychotherapy by specialists in a child guidance clinic. On the other hand, even the non-psychiatric physician may be helpful by giving an individual some insight into why he is reacting as he is and how to deal defensively with stress. As the person talks about his anxiety, he may be relieved from much of it. As he is encouraged to try to meet the stress in a manner which is even partly successful, it may encourage him to take a different position so that in time he will become desensitized. Each success will serve as an encouragement and will reinforce his efforts at attempting to cope. Psychologists using operant conditioning techniques for the relief of fears and other neurotic symptoms base their methods on such an approach.

Since the nature of the child's personality pattern determines to some extent his vulnerability to psychic trauma, and is one of the important elements in predisposing a child to psychosomatic disorders, it is apparent that whatever the physician can do to help an infant and child develop healthy personalities is an important prophylactic step. In molding a child's personality pattern what matters most is the parental attitudes, particularly those of the mother, and her consequent response to the child's needs both for physical and emotional nurture. Hence our attempts earlier in this book to point out ways of enhancing child development through improving mothering and other early child-rearing practices.

A word should be said about the physician's duty to exclude organic disease in those disorders which he believes may be psychosomatic. Certainly an immediate obligation of the physician is to make sure that no serious disorder is being missed and no helpful treatment omitted. This entails careful interviewing and a carefully timed and carefully executed physical examination, along with appropriate and necessary laboratory assessment.

When it is recognized that no primary organic disorder exists, and no treatment is immediately indicated, the physician should make a formal and more complete search for a psychologic disturbance. A real danger exists too many times, when conscientious physicians exaggerate the meaning of somatic symptoms and deal with the patient as if he had an organic illness of specific etiology and known pathology. Overtreatment results and this fosters a denial in the physician and in the patient of psychogenesis. On the other hand, the patient may be more insightful than the physician, raise questions of the psychologic origin and be rebuffed by the physician who either because of disinterest or ignorance prefers not to face psychologic problems.

Without question, some psychogenic disorders become chronic because of the insistence of the physician that they are not psychogenic. When this occurs, invalidism is fostered. This may provide temporary gain to a patient, relieve his symptoms, and seemingly give proof to the physician that his management of the "organic" disorder has been successful. Sooner or later, however, since the basic psychologic difficulties have not been ameliorated, symptoms return, and may be joined by others. The physician must be on his guard lest he misdiagnose this condition as a new illness, or as complications of the previous one. Often parents and patients themselves have by now gained insight, and if courageous enough to mention this to the physician serve as their own diagnostician. When this occurs, it is not enough to expect that they can also heal themselves.

The following case illustrates one pediatric approach to the management of a chronic psychosomatic disorder. It is *not* a complete exposition of ulcerative colitis.

Case of Katy, 13 years old: Ulcerative colitis

Presenting Complaint. Admitted to hospital because of diarrhea of 9 months' duration. At that time while at school she noticed loose stools, and henceforth had 3 to 7 a day with occasional flecks of blood and mucus. She subsequently became anorexic and occasionally had fever as high as 103°F. The diarrhea was not controlled by paregoric.

Six months later the diarrhea increased in intensity and was accompanied by dull, cramping, abdominal pain preceding each diarrheal stool; there were "moderate" amounts of blood in the mucus. She tired easily and menstruation which had started 1 year ago had been absent for 2 months. Examination by sigmoidoscopic study revealed an ulcerated colon. Hemoglobin was 10 grams and she had lost 10 pounds in 3 months. She was admitted to hospital where the diagnosis of ulcerative colitis was verified by local examinations and by x-ray studies. There were no other physical abnormalities detected.

Family. On interviewing the parents it was found that they had been separated for 1 year, were planning a divorce in the near future. There were two younger children, a sister, aged 12 years, and a brother 9. The children were living with the mother but visited the father frequently. The patient was described as being very disturbed about the divorce and the uncertainty as to whom "she should back." She played one parent against the other, tried to manipulate them with the aim of reconciliation. Whenever interviewed, the child appeared anxious, pale, tired easily, and talked of abdominal pain which was aggravated when the talk touched on matters of family.

Treatment. The child was treated with rectal steroid enemas, medication for the anemia and was referred back to the family physician. He saw the child regularly every 2 weeks, regulated the medications and listened sympathetically to the child's talk of her worry about the future. She was able to return to school, did well academically, was esteemed by her peers but described by the teachers as chronically tense and unhappy. Weight gain followed slowly as the diarrhea responded to the drugs. Two months after hospital discharge she was described as being much improved in health generally, had gained 5 pounds in weight, had one formed stool daily without blood.

Her mother and the patient were invited to come to a hospital clinic for presentation to staff. Although each accepted quite willingly, and seemed at ease in the clinical presentation, the child took notice of the remarks of a visiting physician who quite dogmatically gave a bad prognosis. As he predicted that she would have recurrences of colitis, the child was seen to blanche, to turn her head away. She was wheeled out of the amphitheater and began to weep uncontrollably. Attempts at reassurance were made but before leaving the hospital she said that she had to use the bathroom. It was reported by the mother who observed the stool at that time that it contained blood and that the child had severe cramps.

For the next 2 weeks the child had several liquid stools daily with copious bleeding. Her spirit continued to be depressed, she refused to go to school because of fear of soiling and was then referred to a child psychiatrist.

With a combination of psychotherapy, diet and drug regulation, the child slowly regained health so that 18 months after the second episode of diarrhea she was able to face the parental divorce without a recurrence of symptoms or of great emotional distress.

9

A follow-up note from the physician states that menstruation returned and was normal when she was about 15 years old, that her health remained quite good with the exception of occasional bouts of diarrhea with flecking of blood when under special stress. She married at age 20 and delivered a healthy normal infant 12 months later.

From the physician's standpoint, this patient was viewed in a comprehensive manner and the management depended on a combination of physical methods such as diet and drug regulation, and with the modification of emotional and social factors.

Hyperventilation Syndrome

Overbreathing from emotional stress is not uncommon in children 10 years and older. It may occur as a single episode of acute anxiety during a particularly tense life situation, or it may appear frequently when anxiety is chronic. Occasionally it is a manifestation of hysteria.

Although "a breathing difficulty" would be apparent to anyone who is with the child, the patient may be unaware of any respiratory difficulty. The distress is frightening to parents, particularly when it is followed by loss of consciousness, a convulsion or tetany. When the child complains of his discomfort, he may describe it as sensations of choking, shortness of breath, rapidity of respiration, generalized weakness, dizziness, fainting, palpitations and numbness of the hands. The attack may be so unexpected in onset and the symptoms so frightening that the parent reports the first episode promptly to the physician. Where symptoms are less severe but repeated, medical attention may be sought because of their chronicity and invariably because of the "nervousness" of the child.

Parents describe the children as irritable, nervous, rebellious, or as suffering from "tension headaches." When examined by the physician, there is usually no evidence of neurologic disease and no residue of the seizures or tetany. Electroencephalogram findings usually show no disorders, although some show a three-per-second spike and wave during hyperventilation.

The tetany and seizures as well as the syncope which occasionally follows hyperventilation are caused by respiratory alkalosis. Since there are other causes for hyperventilation, particularly intracranial lesions, fever, and drug intoxication (like salicylates), the differential diagnosis must focus on both the immediate physical and emotional conditions, and on the past history and the state of health or disease of the whole body. The paroxysmal nature of the syndrome suggests other periodic disorders; particularly hypotensive syncope, Stokes-Adams disease, epilepsy, migraine, and asthma. Acute anxiety may accompany any of these physical disorders and hence confuse the physician who is looking for a psychogenic factor as being the prime etiologic offender.

The parents are usually concerned lest the condition represent epilepsy. They may be reassured when a thorough and competently done physical examination and an electroencephalogram reveal no signs indicating neurologic disease.

The past history usually indicates that there have been psychologic disturbances in the patient or discord within the family. The non-psychiatric physician can often recognize the precipitating emotional factors and also the reasons for the underlying and chronic anxiety. To help the patient understand the physiologic nature of the symptoms the physician may ask him to overbreathe voluntarily to the point of feeling giddy in order to demonstrate how to rebreathe into a paper bag to terminate the condition. The physician suggests this as the symptomatic treatment for terminating any recurrence of the hyperventilation.

Such suggestion and general reassurance may be effective in helping both child and parent to deal with the symptoms and with some of the superficial stresses. However, in reassuring the patient, the physician should not imply that nothing is wrong. Making light of the symptoms may only give the impression that he is unable to determine the cause of the difficulty.

Sedatives or tranquilizers may be of some benefit during the acute phase of treatment but have no long-term effects. Oxygen is not indicated and may actually intensify the unpleasant symptoms and the underlying anxiety.

Because of the prominence of psychologic factors in the background of the patient and his family the physician's counselling may not be entirely effective and referral to a psychiatric resource is indicated.

When such an evaluation is permitted by the patient and his parents, it is not unusual to find that the child has persistent anxiety, often related to concerns about sexuality, ambivalence towards separating from parents, worry about physical health or an impending operation, and fantasies of death and injury. Sometimes these children are severely depressed, occasionally even schizophrenic.

Chapter 7

PUBERTY AND EARLY ADOLESCENCE
(12 to 15 years)

PUBERTY AND EARLY ADOLESCENCE

Tasks in Process

CHILD

To come to terms with body changes.

To cope with sexual development and psychosexual drives.

To establish and confirm sense of identity.

To learn further re sex role.

To synthesize personality.

To struggle for independence and emancipation from family.

To incorporate learning to the gestalt of living.

PARENT(S)

To help child complete emancipation.

To provide support and understanding.

To limit child's behavior and set standards.

To offer favorable and appropriate environment for healthy development.

To recall own adolescent difficulties; to accept and respect the adolescent's differences or similarities to parents or others.

To relate to adolescents and adolescence with a constructive sense of humor.

Acceptable Behavioral Characteristics

CHILD

Heightened physical power, strength and coordination.

Occasional psychosomatic and somatopsychic disturbances.

Maturing sex characteristics and proclivities.

Review and resolution of oedipal conflicts.

Inconsistent, unpredictable and paradoxical behavior.

Exploration and experimentation with self and world.

Eagerness for peer approval and relationships.

Strong moral and ethical perceptions.

Cognitive development accelerated; deductive and inductive reasoning; operational thought.

Competitive in play; erratic work-play patterns.

Better use of language and other symbolic material.

Critical of self and others; self-evaluative.

Highly ambivalent towards parents.

Anxiety over loss of parental nurturing.

Hostility to parents.

Verbal aggression.

PARENT(S)

Allow and encourage reasonable independence.

Set fair rules; are consistent.

Compassionate and understanding; firm but not punitive or derogatory.

Feel pleasure and pride; occasional guilt and disappointment.

Have other interests besides child.

Marital life fulfilled apart from child.

Occasional expression of intolerance, resentment, envy or anxiety about adolescent's development.

(12 to 15 years)

Minimal Psychopathology

CHILD	PARENT(S)
Apprehensions, fears, guilt and anxiety re sex, health, education.	Sense of failure.
Defiant, negative, impulsive or depressed behavior.	Disappointment greater than joy.
	Indifference to child and family.
Frequent somatic or hypochondriacal complaints; or denial of ordinary illnesses.	Apathy and depression.
	Persistent intolerance of child.
Learning irregular or deficient.	Limited interests and self expression.
Sexual preoccupation.	Loss of perspective about child's capacities.
Poor or absent personal relationships with adults or peers.	Occasional direct or vicarious reversion to adolescent impulses.
Immaturity or precocious behavior; unchanging personality and temperament.	Uncertainty about standards regarding sexual behavior and deviant social or personal activity.
Unwillingness to assume the responsibility of greater autonomy.	
Inability to substitute or postpone gratifications.	

Extreme Psychopathology

CHILD	PARENT(S)
Complete withdrawal into self, extreme depression.	Severe depression and withdrawal.
Acts of delinquency, asceticism, ritualism, over-conformity.	Complete rejection of child and/or family.
	Inability to function in family role.
Neuroses, especially phobias; persistent anxiety, compulsions, inhibitions or constrictive behavior.	Rivalrous, competitive, destructive and abusive to child.
Persistent hypochondriases.	Abetting child's acting out of unacceptable sexual or aggressive impulses for vicarious reasons.
Sex aberrations.	
Somatic illness: anorexia, colitis, menstrual disorders.	Perpetuation of incapacitating infantilism in the pre-adolescent.
Complete inability to socialize or work (learning, etc.)	Panic reactions to acceptable standards of sexual behavior, social activity and assertiveness.
Psychoses.	Compulsive, obsessive or psychotic behavior.

The Complexities of Maturation

The period of physical changes called puberty and its concomitant called adolescence are distinguished by psychologic, social and intellectual changes which are universally recognized as highly significant developmental landmarks.

The adolescent epoch is a normative developmental crisis in which characteristic biologic transformations are accompanied by personality changes. Eruptive psychologic states and capacities usher in the crystallization and synchronization of the more stable biologic and psychologic dynamics of the adult. In contemporary American society the adolescent's tendency to explore and experiment with himself and his world are not channeled into well-defined and institutionalized alternatives. The developmental instabilities of youth in our culture are reflected by how he challenges the options he perceives in his community and by the unrest he evokes in his environment. Known as particularly stressful, a normative and desirable developmental crisis, it is expected that this period of life will produce a variety of problems.

The non-psychiatric physician becomes involved because frequently these problems are manifested first as physical illnesses or as a hypochondriacal attitude. This is a time of increased frequency of psychosomatic and somatopsychic disturbances. It is not to say that severe disturbances are abundant. Most of the problems are normally developmental and transient. However, the physician should be concerned if the adolescent, despite biologic growth and development, is at a standstill in his emotional and temperamental growth. Often this is evidence of constriction and inhibition, which require attention.

In his behavior, for example, it is normal for the adolescent to be paradoxical; to be inconsistent and unpredictable for a considerable length of time. He fights his impulses yet tries to accept them. He uses defenses to ward them off successfully, yet he is overrun by them. As a consequence he loves his parents and hates them, revolts against them, yet remains dependent. It is customary at this time for the adolescent to be deeply ashamed of his parents, unwilling to discuss personal matters with them, but unexpectedly to seek heart-to-heart talks.

As he searches in spurts for his own identity he is both unselfish and self-centered; calculating yet also idealistic and generous. Such fluctuations between extreme opposites would be considered highly abnormal at any other time of life. Now it means nothing more than the lengthy and somewhat explosive transition of emerging adult personality and the continuous experimentation by which it develops.

When illness exists, it is liable to extend into adulthood. This is seen especially in some of the mental illnesses, but is also true for physical sickness like chronic metabolic disorders. For example, adult diabetes is notorious for appearing first in adolescence. Often a thread of development extends backwards too; as when the behavior of the adolescent frequently reflects its origin in earlier experiences.

Adolescence does not spring up suddenly, but is the confluence of many tributaries stemming from physical traits, psychologic characteristics and earlier experiences. How the human organism deals with the most intimate and biologically rooted relationships in infancy and childhood contributes to and shapes the quality of one's life. The theme of parent and child relationship appears as a particularly poignant one in adolescence. For example, the role of father as creator, protector and mentor begins to be challenged by the son in adolescence. As each struggles with his emotions, the one to maintain his manhood and the other to show his readiness for attaining it, intense and universal feelings of life are involved. Feelings of love, fear, admiration, rivalry, hostility, rejection, pride and guilt may be expressed directly and openly or in disguise. In either case, they often bring parent and child to the physician as the conflict intensifies. Mother and daughter have similar interests and conflicts which are related to the oedipal relationships first established in the pre-school age. The daughter tests her femininity in rivalry for the father's affection. Yet she is ambiguous and chary about her developing female role and conflictive with her mother about achieving it.

For better or worse we have no myths or rituals in our society to help a child effectively make the transition from childhood through adolescence and to help him confirm his identity. Instead, the turbulence of this age period is a baptism under fire, and while painful for all parties concerned, it typically initiates the adolescent. In fact, we often worry if the dramatic biologic changes are not accompanied by exploratory erratic behavior indicating that inner changes are being expressed socially and adequately. Although experimental, rebellious behavior makes the adolescent a difficult member of his family and neighborhood, an ascetic, excessively controlled or withdrawn adolescent is much less likely to attain the mature stability and capacities of a healthy adulthood.

Sexual Development

The stress of the period arises from the child's attempts to accomplish several goals. He must deal with the changes of his body, and the effects of these on his performance. Intricate changes in muscles, bones and joints at first cause awkwardness. The child's sensitiveness to this is acute, despite improvement in physical strength, vigor and prowess. If he can believe that improved coordination will also follow, he will be less prone to be self-critical and avoid fanatically practicing his skills, or to feel inferior in comparison to his peers.

The appearance of secondary sex characteristics, changes in size of the sex organs in boys and the beginning of menstruation in girls are accompanied by increased pleasurable sensations of sexuality. Coping with these strong psychosexual drives involves the adolescent in conflicts and in attitudes about sex which he has learned and adopted from his parents. In his attempts to adapt, he may feel anxiety and guilt. These emotions in turn produce a variety of behavior, from extreme inhibition and denial to acting-out experimentation. This may take the form of temporary homosexual and heterosexual activities, or to increased masturbation. Anxiety and guilt may be heightened further by such activities.

In boys the range of usual homosexuality in adolescence extends from sex play in locker rooms and school lavatories and grabbing of each other's genitals, to single episodes of experimentation with mutual masturbation. None of these transient practices preclude normal progress to heterosexuality.

One type of homosexual relationship that boys do not allow themselves is experimentation in sexual acts with grown men. Even delinquent boys have strict taboos about such relationships. Newspapers frequently carry items about a boy or a group of adolescents attacking a man who proposed a homosexual relationship with one of them. Guilt feelings about homosexuality may be assuaged by their hostility and even murderous acts against a homosexual man who has made advances. When a boy repeats sexual practices with other males and in time takes the role of the seducer, homosexuality is no longer considered developmentally normal, but must be viewed as a psychopathologic condition. Competent psychotherapy utilized early may help a boy overcome the practice and help him advance to normal heterosexuality.

Girls show much less unmodified homosexual license; overt activity is infrequent and when it appears, it involves a pair of girls more than a group. Furtive homosexual games between partners is occasionally reported as breast play or mutual masturbation.

A boy despite anxiety and considerable guilt is willing to take risks. Girls may develop crushes for each other but also show greater prohibition along with guilt and anxiety although they feel freer to kiss and embrace each other casually than do boys. For some, even these customary acts of friendship are frightening and a relationship may be terminated because it suddenly appears to be dangerous. Quite common among girls is a morbid dread of body contact with other girls and women, and an expression of disgust and loathing towards women and women's bodies may occur in its most virulent form against the mother herself. Apparently, homosexuality represents for the girl a dangerous regression to a more dependent relationship.

The swing in our culture from restrictive social attitudes to the more permissive is seen in the changes of many middle- and upper-class parents. Greater emphasis on children's participation in social activities such as dating and partying earlier in life, as well as exposing them to cocktail parties with loose talk of sex, has contributed to premature and excessive sex excitation. It is difficult enough for most adolescents to control and sublimate their sex feelings. Enforcing early sociability helps provoke promiscuity and asocial behavior. Parents of adolescents still belong on the controlling side until such time as the adolescent's maturity permits self-control and responsibility.

Helpful Guidance

What parents do in such matters as making rules will further influence the adolescent's reactions. Parents and professional persons are often perplexed as to what to do. Their apparent anxiety and vacillation is upsetting to the child who hoped to find in them constancy and consistency. The vacillating parent hesitates to take a strong position with the child lest he be considered unfair or punitive, and often mistakes the child's rebelliousness and criticisms as evidence of parental failure or inability to make correct decisions. Actually, the adolescent frequently is projecting feelings of resentment against himself onto the parent. Aware of his own conflict and difficulty in making decisions and setting rules of discipline, he makes it appear as if the parent represented one side of his conflict and feelings which he then opposes. One often witnesses this kind of reaction in a child who argues with a parent against a curfew, yet is desirous of having a parent set such limits for him. In the eyes of peers it is much more acceptable to blame parents for their lack of understanding about when to come home at night than to bear the responsibility himself.

The physician often can help the adolescent when asked for guidance in personal decision-making regarding dating and sexual behavior. Speaking as a mature professional person without moralizing one may help adolescents weigh values and morals with the understanding that ultimately the decision rests on the young person.

Adolescence is a time of much re-evaluation of the self physically, emotionally, socially and ethically. The teen-ager is severely critical of himself, as well as of others. He feels guilty about many things. This may turn him to religion. His interest may be sporadic, but it is real and intense. He has ethical and moral concerns, and fights for justice. The interest in religion may lead to asceticism, to withdrawal from the world. Such behavior may border on the psychotic, but withdrawal from others may change suddenly and completely, as if social exchange with peers is safe again. The adolescent finds association with peers reassuring and comforting for the most part, especially when they accept him as one of their own kind. While he wants to be different, yet he also hopes to be like his peers. He tries to conform, and may protect himself by over-conforming to the standards and behavior of peers as well as of parents.

In much that he does, the adolescent seeks affirmation of his self and confirmation of his new identifications. He needs opportunity to establish his identity, and to learn how to be himself sexually and socially. If he cannot find himself as an individual, as a member of his peer group and as a contributing member of society, he often develops symptoms. Learning, which normally spurts in this period of life, especially in inductive and deductive reasoning and in operational thought, may become irregular and inhibited. He may become defiant of parents and other authority and behave in a delinquent or alienated manner. He may develop a serious work or study inhibition or illness. Some of the extreme problems brought to the attention of the physician appear in Chapter 11.

The role of the parents and their tasks have been alluded to in describing the nature of the adolescent. In principle they are similar to those assumed earlier in the life of the child. Most prominent is assistance with his struggles for independence. Most parents understand the need to help a child emancipate himself completely but they have mixed feelings about this. On the one hand, they feel that there is little they can do, that nature will take its course. On the other hand, they feel they still need to exert control because the adolescent seems so adult in his impulses and yet so incapable and unready for self-determination and self-control. A parent may see his own adolescent strivings and problems re-enacted in his child and this adds to his uneasiness. They may fear that "the evil one does lives after him" and that their inability to control the adolescent represents a threat against the control of their own middle-aged impulses.

Often parents find fault and are critical with their own rearing methods. They struggle to improve on methods which they learned from their own parents. Most parents are pleased, even relieved, when their child assumes greater independence and requires less control. There is even some pride in his accomplishments. But often there is also disappointment in his efforts. For example, attainment in school may not be what was expected despite the opportunities provided. The child's athletic prowess may not compare with what the father expected and he himself attained. The choice of a career, even to the extent of schooling, may give the parents the feeling that they have failed in motivating their child sufficiently. Often this is expressed as an intense resentment that the child has been "spoiled" and is ungrateful. If his influence is to be effective, the physician must create tolerance by the parents for the teen-ager's assertion of unique independence and self-realization even if it does not conform to their notions of what form and substance this goal should become.

The physician can frequently help parents deal with their own hurt pride, disappointment and guilt by listening and pointing out that their efforts necessarily do not represent failure or "bad parentage." They should be advised not to reject those adolescents whom they find wanting, but rather to try to enjoy their differences and their efforts to establish their own careers.

Some parents, particularly mothers, become depressed during the adolescence of their children. It points out to them their own aging, and displacement by what seems a beautiful, healthier, more successful and young generation. Feelings caused by the menopause as well as those stemming from the strained relationships to their children, and sometimes to their husband, can induce a depression.

The physician performs an important service to parents when he helps them prepare for these later years long before their children begin adolescence. A mother who already begins to find interests other than those of family when the child is of school age may be protecting herself against a difficult period later on. Pointing out to parents the need for fulfilling their lives with each other is within the realm of good medical guidance.

The adolescent is not the only one who needs sex education; his parents are also in need, not only for preparing themselves to deal with their growing children, but with their own sexual feelings and sexual roles. Too often parents lose their sexual attractiveness for each other, and diagnose their frigidity and impotence as evidence of aging. Usually it is not that at all; the cause is primarily a psychologic one.

As has been mentioned before, parents serve as models for identification, for objects of positive and negative imitation in most matters of behavior beginning in infancy. In adolescence, parents continue to be models, especially as marriage partners. Parents who mutually respect each other, who continue to be tender and affectionate with each other, offer the best models for identification, setting standards which the adolescent unwittingly will try to achieve.

Fears

As a rule, adolescents do not come to a physician with an outright request for help with their fears, although basically they are fearful. But frequently they become involved in situations which bring about referral by others. The fears may relate to growing up, or to meeting new experiences like facing a new peer group, going to camp, promotion in school, or taking a first job. In later adolescence such fears are precipitated by going away to college, to take a job or to serve in a military capacity.

Like adolescence itself, fears may emerge with relevance to earlier unresolved difficulties and tensions. The fears of childhood such as of the dark, or insistence that the bedroom door remain open, or of physical injury, may continue in only slightly modified form from childhood. Then again they may convert to what seems like more age-appropriate representations, such as requiring the sound of a radio if the door is closed, or refusal to engage in sports to camouflage fear of physical injury.

In adolescence the child may be somewhat more sophisticated about concealing his fears than he was in childhood, but they may exact their toll in behavioral aberrations or in somatopsychic manifestations. Often negativism and behavior which parents may find inexplicable stem from unexpressed fears. When parents astutely perceive the underlying fear and give voice to it, the adolescent's defenses spur him to vehement denial. It is difficult for the parent and even the physician to bring the adolescent to "talk it out" but if the physician in the course of examination can obliquely refer to typical human fears and apprehensions, the adolescent may respond to such discussion and even become subjective. It should be underscored that the difficulty in acknowledging these fears and worries reflects the adolescent's increased uncertainty about his self-control, his fate, and what is perceived as the magic power of a thought or strong emotion. He reacts as though verbalization of the unacceptable fearsome thought or feeling will cause it to take place in the most permanent and damaging way. The danger of mental "magic" is reduced significantly when the adolescent and doctor can find a tolerable way to let awareness, verbalization and ventilation take place.

Case of Nancy N., age 15 years: Fear of sex and death

History. Nancy had been referred to a pediatric clinic at the age of 10 for allergic rhinitis. Over the years she had received a variety of medicine and other treatment. In the past year she had returned to the clinic regularly at 1- or 2-week intervals for antigen injections. Despite the discomfort of the needles and the time lost from other activities to come to the clinic, it was apparent that she enjoyed her visits and became dependent on them. At one point placebo injections were given instead of the regular antigens, and gave her as much relief.

The pediatrician recognized her dependence on him and began to inquire into her background. He found that her father had died when she was 9 years old, and that it was difficult to talk about this because she and her mother continued to grieve and talked much about him. It was an Italian Catholic family, closely knit. Mother and daughter lived on Social Security benefits. There were two younger siblings.

Nancy was a small, attractive girl who looked younger than her age. She talked rapidly and dramatically, and tried to give the impression of continual gaiety and happiness. She worked hard at her parochial high school work but was unable to keep up with the college preparatory courses. She decided on a secretarial career. She had few friends, and they were usually younger than she. She had one "pen-pal," a member of a professional ice skating team. She had also formed a close association with the priest in her parish, and was fond of a teacher in the high school and had fantasies about marrying him. In the last year she began to have dates, went to parties, but when the lights were turned off and kissing games began she became frightened, sick to her stomach, and had to leave the party.

In further interviews, the girl confided that she hoped never to grow up, because this involved relationships with men and these could be dangerous. For example, they could die, such as her father had done; or they could be too "sexy." She talked about her fears of getting involved sexually, of becoming pregnant, yet she had little accurate knowledge about sexual development and behavior.

Course and Management. Her attending physician left the community, so it was necessary to refer her to another. This was a good step, since she had already become too dependent on him. The new physician planned to help her wean herself from the clinic, and from medical treatment, as a step in developing an image of herself as a healthy adolescent rather than as a sickly younger child. They were able to talk about sexual matters, physical development, intercourse and pregnancy. It was pointed out that death of a parent was less common than she believed; that childbirth was not to be feared. Appointments to the clinic were made infrequent, and all injections ceased. With the patient's permission the physician talked with her priest about Nancy's guilt around sex and sin.

The priest was an enlightened young man who did not hold with the concept that masturbation was sinful. He agreed to recommend to Nancy that she attend a new course on sex which was given by a specialist in adolescent medicine.

In a letter several months later Nancy reported that she had been promoted in school, was dating more or less steadily a young man of similar racial and religious background, that she looked forward to going to a secretarial school and to marrying.

Hypochondriasis and Fatigability

Preoccupation with bodily sensations, and thoughts of illness and fatigue are frequent among adolescents. The diagnosis of hypochondriasis is made when the physician after careful physical assessment finds no disease. If the physician seeks further, he will usually find symptoms of anxiety and phobias, which the patient interprets as physical disease. For example, palpitation, overbreathing (see Hyperventilation Syndrome p. 116), a jitteriness called "nervousness" are frequent complaints.

While it is true that the adolescent tires easily, and has reason to be fatigued because of the kind of life he leads, his organism is remarkably resilient and sturdy. Therefore, chronic fatigue, oversleeping in the morning and failing to keep appointments, resorting to bed frequently during the daytime hours, are symptoms of an emotional upset, sometimes genuine depressions. Tiredness may be an unconscious defense which gives temporary gain but in the long run works to the detriment of the adolescent. If the condition is recognized for what it is, and management directed not only toward alleviating the symptom, but also at the basic problem, much immediate benefit will come to the teenager and will also help to prevent future trouble. Some adolescents are never able to give up behavior which brings them certain gratification, even if unhealthy. Later they tend to resort to chronic invalidism as a way of coping with the problems of adulthood as well.

Unfortunately, some physicians consider such a patient as an immature individual who could snap out of it if he really wanted to. If the physician will extend himself to look beyond the complaints, spend time listening to the patient and getting him to talk about himself, it is frequently found that the adolescent has good reason to feel miserable. Not only are the sensations real, but the causative emotional states are genuine. The patient may be depressed, occasionally schizophrenic. The physician's responsibility is to rule out physical disease, but having done that once, not to continue unnecessary studies. Overtreatment is also to be avoided. Some of the psychotherapeutic measures which help these adolescents include support, reassurance, providing insight, and others (See chapter 9 on Management).

Case of Peter R.: Genesis of hypochondriasis

The older of two children and only son of a middle-class Jewish family, Peter was doted on by his devoted family including the grandparents. During the earlier years the pediatrician had encouraged the parents to consider Peter as the vigorous healthy boy that he was. However, the mother's migraine headaches and a serious lung infection suffered by Peter's sister as an infant had created an atmosphere of great apprehensiveness about the children's health. Peter began to sustain a moderate hypochondriasis which represented the convergence of his special meaning to the family, an identification with his adoring and adored mother, and the fear that he would also be as critically ill as his sister had been.

When he was 12 years old, the physician recommended that Peter be encouraged to join the neighborhood scout troop, and at 13 years of age he supported the boy's interest in camping and in having a 2-weeks' summer camp experience. The physician examined him and answered his questions about the risk of poison ivy, what to do about constipation and headaches. Then he explained to the boy that he had a strong body and sound health. The camp experience confirmed the diagnosis. As Peter's development progressed, the hypochondriasis disappeared. In later years the young man dated his "good" health as having begun simultaneously with his camp experience.

The physician in reviewing his patient's development indicated that it was not until the boy was old enough to trust his own critical faculties and to assert beginning independent strivings that the doctor's attitude of a strong body and sound health was taken over by Peter as his own attitude.

Conversion Reactions

Children like adults may deal with emotional conflicts by unconsciously repressing them. A further consequence is the conversion of the strong emotions with symbolic significance into psychosomatic dysfunction, involving a disturbance of parts and organs of the body supplied by the voluntary portion of the central nervous system. The striated muscles and the somatosensory apparatus are ordinarily involved.

Conversion disorders produce a variety of symptoms. The most frequent include disturbances in motor function as in paralysis or motor tics, alterations in sensory perception as in blindness or deafness, disturbances in awareness as in syncope or convulsion-like phenomena. The gastrointestinal tract may be involved producing symptoms of vomiting or encopresis; the respiratory tract when affected responds with hyperventilation, respiratory tics. There may also be bladder symptoms, particularly frequency of urination and enuresis. Sometimes unusual combinations of symptoms occur which resemble a psychosis.

The symptoms symbolize emotional conflict which assumes the form of illness and suffering. Frequently this provides unconscious secondary gains resulting from the increased dependence on other persons, especially parents. Anxiety is at the base of the conflict although this may not be consciously acknowledged. The psychologic determinants of the symptoms vary, but it is not unusual for a child to identify with the symptom of a parent. Some psychiatrists feel that such symptoms are learned, in fact that the whole neurotic pattern has been learned and hence should

10

be treated by techniques which help the patient unlearn, or at least become desensitized to the basic anxiety. It is difficult to understand how some of these symptoms are gainful to the patient, particularly when they seem to produce so much pain and discomfort. In such instances, secondary gain arises from the unconscious need for punishment.

Transient conversion symptoms may appear in reactions to specific situational stresses in children, particularly during convalescence from physical illness. Persons whose body parts are immobilized as in traction or by casts may have fantasies and complain of symptoms which could not possibly follow anatomic lines or physiologic processes.

Typical is the patient who complains that his leg immobilized in the cast nevertheless "bends as in walking." Or a child's naive concept of bodily function may lead to his description of functions of the gastro-intestinal tract which are impossible. An adolescent who has had a partial resection of the bowel, and grasps this concept intellectually, nevertheless describes pain in those parts which no longer are present. Adolescents who have had eye surgery, and who have recovered from all dysfunction, nevertheless may continue to complain as if the illness still existed.

In adolescents as in adults, conversion disorders frequently occur in hysterical personalities, most common in females but occasionally appearing also in males. The disability may be present constantly, without remission or interruption, or intermittently, and is resistant to specific treatment until such time when it no longer serves the purpose of the patient or yields to interpretive psychotherapy motivated by the suffering caused by this illness.

Although the physician may suspect the psychogenic etiology, each of these patients should be given a thorough physical, and particularly a neurologic examination. Since hearing and visual defects are frequently first diagnosed in adolescence, every adolescent should have thorough hearing and vision tests.

When the diagnosis of conversion disorder is made, the physician should explain to the patient and his parents that the patient has a strong body and that no physical disease exists. The doctor should not imply that symptoms are without meaning or are unreal. The fact that the causative agent has a psychologic base should be explained carefully, since it is difficult for many people to comprehend. Often, the more sophisticated parent will raise the question of psychogenesis when told that no physical disease exists. The patient should never be criticized or condemned for what has come about unconsciously. He needs help in getting insight into the emotional nature of the problem, and then assistance in dealing with his conflicts so that healthier psychologic mechanisms may be invoked in coping with his difficulties.

Conversion symptoms if treated palliatively become more difficult to cure. Overtreatment should be avoided also. The repeating of laboratory tests and x-rays simply to convince the patient and his parents that he has no physical illness may only confirm the patient's belief that he is so afflicted, despite the physician's verbal reassurance that the problem is psychologic. Using drugs or other measures to treat conversion symptoms as if they were indeed the effects of a physical illness may temporarily help the patient. The suggestive force of the measures may cause the symptoms to disappear, only to return later requiring further medical management. Recurrences are not unusual under such a regimen.

It is important that the parents be told that the child is not imagining an illness, nor malingering but that he is truly suffering from symptoms of an emotional disturbance. Investigation of the emotional stresses in the child's life, noting the interpersonal and the transactional relationships with parents and peers in home and school, frequently give patient and physician clues to the bases of stress. Suggestion or reassurance alone are not enough in helping the child. Firm but understanding insistence that the child resume his responsibilities, gradually leave his bed, try to use the affected part of the body and enter the mainstream of life is always indicated. For the child who is particularly tense and has trouble relaxing, prescriptions may be given for simple exercises, not with the idea of overcoming a physical deficiency, but rather for helping him to overcome the emotional tension which is basic to the symptoms. Hypnosis as a rule has only temporary benefit and should never be carried out except by persons carefully trained and experienced in its use.

Conversion symptoms as well as hysterical reactions which have been present for a long time cannot be handled psychologically by a non-psychiatric physician. His role continues to be that of supervising the general physical health of the patient.

Anxiety Reactions

These are characterized by apprehension, fearfulness, and tension not necessarily related to any particular situation or object. It is normal for every person to experience acute or chronic anxiety reactions. The former comes on quickly, lasts for a few minutes or several hours, and seems unrelated to any event in contrast to fears, which are frequently connected with some experience such as going to school, entering a hospital and so on. In chronic anxiety the tenseness and the apprehension may last for weeks and months and sometimes longer. The adolescent frequently describes anxiety when he complains of nervousness, tension or panic. Separation anxiety has already been described as typical and normal in infancy and around times of entering school. Anxiety reactions seem particularly common in early adolescence and increase in clinical frequency from then on into early adulthood as new experiences are faced in making decisions about schools, work and sexual relationship.

Acute Anxiety

The adolescent with an acute anxiety reaction feels a sudden fearfulness as if something bad were about to happen to him. He may become agitated and complain of physical sensations like dizziness, headache, and migraine. There may be nausea and vomiting. Comforting by a parent may put a temporary end to the attack, but recurrences are common and soon may present a clue as they follow the same type of stressful situation. The physician frequently is consulted for the physical signs and symptoms, but rather easily is able to rule out physical disease after obtaining a careful history of the problem, talking with the child and parents, and doing a physical examination. The physician who is convinced of the true nature of the difficulty, can show his confidence in his examination by telling the parents that the child's anxiousness is not induced by physical disease but is related to stress and to conflicts about personal feelings, longings and self-criticism. The lay term "nervousness" is inappropriate, although it continues to be in common use and has some value in describing the feelings of the patient. Too often, however, parents are unable to accept that diagnosis, feel it is a reflection of their own care and rearing and shop around for evidence to prove that the diagnosis is not correct. They would prefer a chemical or metabolic disorder easily treated with drugs and they may press physicians for such medications. Obviously, no physician should be caught in that trap because it only leads to disillusionment and ultimately to the severance of the relationship with the patient. This does not mean that sedatives are always contraindicated. Sometimes the anxiety reactions are so great and severe, sleeplessness so long continued that parents and child have secondary symptoms related to fatigue. But the medications should be used to provide relief and not as agents which are expected miraculously to remove the basic emotional components of the anxiety reactions. Adolescents may become addicted to the use of drugs such as barbiturates and other sedatives just as they may become habituated to a life of semi-invalidism and overprotection.

In general, the non-psychiatric physician can deal adequately with many cases of acute anxiety. When the symptoms are not severe nor longstanding, and when the parents and adolescent are cooperative and willing to talk about stresses and conflicts in their lives, psychotherapeutic assistance is invoked effectively and tactfully without the physician being actually aware of it. The more he knows about the psychologic management of anxiety, the better he is able to help his patient overcome his difficulties. Should he not have the time, experience or knowledge he should refer the adolescent and his parents to other professional persons such as psychiatrists, child guidance clinics and family counselling services.

Case of Ann, aged 13 years: Acute generalized anxiety

Present History. Ann had been in a minor automobile accident, had escaped unhurt, but was upset because she had been interrogated by the police as a witness. Although she dramatically gave an account of the accident to her mother that evening, it seemed not to be important. However 1 month later, on a day when Ann was to take part in a school play, she refused to enter the bus which usually picked her up each morning. Although she could not explain clearly why she feared entering the bus, she described feelings of impending death; the poor ventilation of the bus always gave her feelings of "smelly substances" and the fear that she would pick up a disease. The rest of the day she seemed without discomfort but refused to leave the house. That night she had a nightmare which she could not describe. The following day she entered the bus on urging by the mother but stopped the driver after one mile, to be let out because she "couldn't breathe." Although she continued to feel that way, she was able to walk home and sit comfortably as she talked to her mother about the lack of safety of automobiles, the high death rate from traffic accidents, and her fantasy that she would one day succumb to one of them. The respiratory difficulty continued for several hours. That evening a physician was called.

On examination Ann was hyperventilating, appeared shy and resistant to undressing, but as far as could be determined she was not physically sick. Diagnosis of acute anxiety was made to the child and to the mother and the question was raised about the reasons for her newly acquired fear of automobiles. Appointment was made for the physician in his office 3 days hence. It was kept, but the child walked the distance of 3 miles rather than come by auto.

She seemed healthy, cooperative, not very talkative and somewhat distrusting. The family history was inquired into and it was found that the father had left the family, that a divorce was pending, that the three children of the family, one older than Ann and one younger, accused the mother of unwillingness to try to bring the husband back into the family. He had left on the mother's insistence because he was gambling, did not bring in enough money to support the family and this had forced the mother to work part time.

Beginning with her birth Ann's early life had been uneventful. She had always been considered an unnaturally quiet and good baby, there had been no pre-school difficulties, and the child's work in grammar school was moderately well done. In retrospect Mrs. M. thought that Ann had become somewhat quieter in the preceding months, lazier, dirty and no longer willing to do her share of the household work. She had recently become interested in boys and a neighbor had reported that Ann and her son had been found fondling the genitals of each other while alone in the basement. Although the mother had not talked about birth and pregnancy to her daughter, she had briefly talked about menstruation which had started at age 12 years.

In the office interview with the physician Ann expressed unwillingness to return to school by bus or to travel in any auto, but did agree to walk on a highway with rather heavy traffic. She was encouraged to do this and the mother reported the following day that return to school had been accomplished successfully. That evening, Ann had spent an unusually long time in the bathroom and the mother accused her of masturbating. The child denied this, wept, became abusive, and complained of difficulty with breathing and a fear of death. The physician made a house call, talked to the patient, tried to reassure her that there was no physical disorder, and asked that the mother stop accusing the daughter about her sexual behavior. Referral was made to a child guidance clinic in the community and the first appointment was held the following day because the matter seemed urgently in need of attention.

Child Guidance Clinic Evaluation. The child guidance appraisal consisted of trying to determine the child's feelings and attitudes about many things. It was apparent that she was misinformed and frightened about sex. She admitted petting with a boyfriend on numerous occasions, masturbation by self and with her sisters, and considered much of this sinful because her mother had labeled it so. She believed that she had sinned and must make atonement, but could not find a way which seemed satisfactory; daily church attendance was unsatisfactory as penance. After eight interviews with Ann alone, and three interviews with the mother, the child was reconciled to the fact that what she was doing was not sinful or abnormal, that no penance was required, and that it was unlikely that she would suffer any harmful consequences directly or indirectly because of her interest in sexual matters or because of what she had done sexually. During the time that she came to the child guidance clinic, there were occasional periods of breathlessness when she talked about matters which disturbed her, but she was never so "nervous" that she could not go to school nor compete satisfactorily there. The acute anxiety was relieved but the underlying psychological difficulties which came to light through the expression of this anxiety required more attention.

Chronic Anxiety

Much that has been said before also applies to these conditions. They frequently result from acute anxiety which has not been resolved. The reason for this may be that the crisis or the factors leading to the disorder were so repetitive and so chronic as stimulating agents that the child's ability to cope with them failed although he may have been quite successful with lesser problems. Although the anxiety frequently stems from difficulties in interpersonal relationships, the basic causes relate to conflicts between the sexual and aggressive drives and the controlling mechanisms of the ego and superego. Feelings, thoughts and attitudes are repressed, guilt is felt consciously, defensive mechanisms are invoked unconsciously and anxiety is one of the products.

An important difference between the anxiety reactions of the adolescent and the adult is its immediate relevancy to the causative and precipitating factors. Hence, attempts at intervention and amelioration are potentially more successful with the adolescent. Since the interpersonal causes of his tension are more apparent they are more available for modification by working with parents, the adolescent and others in the community who may be involved. Adolescents with chronic anxiety are prone to complain of symptoms referable to the gastrointestinal and respiratory tracts, and the head and neck. Pains, aches, diarrhea, shortness of breath, muscle tension, visual and hearing difficulties, along with fatigue, are prominent.

The role of the physician is not so much to treat the symptom as to understand the meaning of the complaints, and to inquire into the child's interpersonal relationships and other problems with which the adolescent is attempting to deal. Labelling a condition as nervousness, spastic bowel, growing pains, or a rundown condition is not only misleading but potentially harmful because it emphasizes the possibility of a physical disease and disregards the emotional components. The symptoms may require treatment but this should be no substitute for concern with general health and management of the whole patient. Hospitalization is rarely indicated for the study and treatment of the anxious patient. Where the anxiety has led to chronicity of symptoms because of sustained associated physical illness, hospitalization may be indicated but if carried out, the physician should realize that this experience in itself may be anxiety-provoking.

Anorexia Nervosa (Psychogenic Malnutrition; Gastrointestinal Hysteria)

Although this condition may appear in pre-pubertal children, it is more commonly found in adolescents, particularly females. It seems related to the conflict over growing up and assuming an adult role, sexually and otherwise. It is a psychophysiologic disorder not ascribed to one single type of neurosis. Frequently it appears as a compulsive reaction, or as an accompaniment of hysteria, a depression, or schizophrenia.

Generally there is a history of early struggle between child and parents over feeding and being fed. In adolescence it is reactivated in rejection of food as a means of postponing maturation, especially of femininity. Occasionally a patient is able to provide a clue to the psychogenic etiology by saying, "I cannot stomach what my parents want me to do. I feel they are always pushing something down my throat." Anger and defiance are passively expressed in the refusal to eat. The negativism is intensified when there is parental entreaty to take more food. This illness has important secondary gains as a way out of a developmental crisis and as a means of compelling others to display attention, solicitude and love.

In a sense, anorexia nervosa is misnamed, since anorexia is not a prominent early symptom and may never be one. The disorder follows a period of food rejection or food eaten is vomited by self-induced gagging to a point where there is extreme weight loss. Some patients do not hide their vomiting, but seem to take particular pleasure in retaliating against a mother by vomiting food which she has taken great pains to prepare. This behavior is often accompanied by exaggerated interest in foods and in cooking. There may also be ingestion of huge amounts of particular foodstuffs, such as carbohydrates and odd combinations of foods. For example, charred toast mixed with dried cottage cheese, heavily flavored with salt, ketchup and spiced pickles may be highly preferred.

Parental concern may first be expressed over the peculiar eating habits or food interests and then over the evident weight loss. Concomitant with this history, there often is restlessness, as well as overexercise with the intent to lose weight. Many of these girls place themselves on restricted diets in order to control their weight, either because they were obese or because they considered themselves too heavy, equating the feminine adult figure with excessive weight.

Amenorrhea, constipation, complaints about feeling cold are accompanying symptoms. None of these however seem to worry the patient who gloats over the fact that her weight continues to decline. There is a lowered basal metabolic rate, low blood pressure, a bradycardia, and sooner or later an anemia and a depression of the number of white blood cells. As a consequence of the latter, there is a predisposition to infections of the respiratory tract and of buccal mucous membranes.

This psychogenic condition is more common today than one realizes. Often it appears in a less overt form than described above. Many young women, who are narcissistically proud of their figures, their slimness, and their ability to lose weight, are actually suffering from this disorder. While seductive, they may be disinclined to have dates with boys, and seem disinterested in marriage. Intellectually they are mentally alert, bright, their work habits frequently are obsessive and perfectionistic. They often are considered competent employees.

The diagnosis may be perplexing when there is relatively little loss of appetite and no seeming reduction in caloric intake. At the onset when the symptoms are mild, it does not appear to be a psychiatric condition. However, the psychopathologic situation is clearly evident when there is a constellation of symptoms. Psychiatrists treating such patients often find resistance to therapy at the beginning. When the patient's confidence is won, however, she usually confides to him her hostility to parents, fear of sexual aggression (particularly oral impregnation through kissing), guilt over masturbation, and a drive for perfectionism and success as a defense against her envy of persons of the opposite sex.

In addition to suggesting psychiatric treatment, and usually before doing so, the role of the non-psychiatrist is to preserve life and restore physiologic homeostasis. Hospitalization may well be indicated not only to assess the condition of the patient, administer fluids and start an appropriate feeding regimen, including tube feeding if necessary, but also to separate the child from parents and home. Despite seeming resistance, adolescents often welcome the opportunity to enter hospital and abandon the defense mechanisms which are more or less self-destructive. Initial negativism is soon replaced by confidence in the control by the physician and other staff members. Close liaison between staff members is required to combat successfully the patient's drive to lose weight. Overall management should be guided by psychiatric principles and usually should include formal psychotherapy.

Prognosis depends on the nature of the underlying psychiatric disturbance. For the younger child with a shorter duration of the illness there is a better prognosis. Parents should be involved in all psychotherapy not only to be kept informed and aware of what lies ahead, but to be helped to reorganize their relationship with the child. They need to learn how to help their child assume more independent roles and develop self-esteem. They need help to overcome their solicitous attitude about diet and feeding.

Patients and parents are equally filled with guilt about their relationships to each other, and these feelings need to be faced with the psychotherapist. The child should be reassured that his ambivalent feelings about growing up and independence from parents are not wrong, that hostility, one of the normal mechanisms of parents and children in their attempts to emancipate the relationships, can be controlled and respected. Parents need to be helped to see that they have not failed and that faulty rearing habits in early childhood have not "marked" their children for all time with a neurosis. They should be reassured that the human body is resilient, that every parent makes mistakes, and there are no guaranteed guidelines in child-rearing which produce perfect adults.

Ultimately the prognosis depends on the nature of the psychologic conflict, the patient's individual personality, the insight gained by all parties concerned and the combined skill of pediatricians, psychiatrists, and other hospital staff members.

Menstrual Disorders

Irregularity of the menses is common in the first several months after its onset. This is probably because the cycles are anovulatory. Concern may be minimized if mothers are reminded of this physiologic state and correctly interpret it to the child who is learning about menstruation. Those who suffer irregularities may be readily reassured when given knowledge about the reasons.

Excessive menstrual flow is not uncommon in adolescents, and in younger girls it is likely to be acyclic. When it occurs, it causes fatigue and considerable anxiety. Because it is likely that the production of progesterone is low, prompt appropriate endocrine and psychologic therapy usually brings about a normal flow. In view of the importance of a girl's attitude towards later assuming an adult feminine role, recognition both of her feelings and also the probable physiologic basis of her complaint is essential.

Amenorrhea. Some girls with a normal menstrual history for the first few months or years may gradually or suddenly stop menstruating. In mild forms this is called "boarding school amenorrhea." It often follows anxiety and tension about starting new experiences such as entering schools. Graduate students in colleges are frequently afflicted. Normality of flow may be resumed after reassurance that there is no physical illness involved. The problem may again recur with new concerns about such items as passing grades or acceptance to a club and peer group. Where a girl is not reassured, as when with persistence she incorrectly believes that she is pregnant, the amenorrhea tends to continue so long as the worry is present.

Amenorrhea of a more serious nature is that found in anorexia nervosa

(See page 138). Such amenorrhea, without demonstrable organic disease, usually carries with it a history of acute psychologic stress even though some children show no evidence of emotional trauma. The majority are dependent, insecure, docile and well-behaved. It is difficult for parents to understand that these commendable attributes are excessive and contribute to the patient's emotional distress. As in anorexia nervosa, psychotherapy may be indicated even in the milder cases of amenorrhea without organic disease.

Since a pelvic examination is indicated in all of these individuals, the physician who undertakes it should realize that such an examination to the uninformed adolescent may be anxiety-provoking as well as painful. It should be deferred until the confidence of the patient has been won, and time has permitted an explanation about the indications for and the techniques of pelvic examination. It goes without saying that gentleness and lack of force must be employed as well as regard for the dignity and the privacy of the patient, even more than if she were an adult.

The examination should be made by a skilled gynecologist assisted by a nurse to avoid unnecessary re-examinations especially where there may be equivocal findings. An examination which is done crudely and inexpertly not only fails to provide information, but is pain producing. For the child who has been taught that it is wrong to handle the genitals, an insertion of an instrument or the fingers into the vagina may embarrass or frighten the young female. Rarely does she find the experience erotically pleasurable.

Psychologic consideration should accompany endocrine studies after the thorough physical examination has ruled out organic disease. Endocrine therapy directed towards restoration of menstrual cycles and ovulation reassures the parents and the patient, except in those instances where the adolescent rejects her feminine role.

Improvement in nutrition, and in hormonal and metabolic physiology, is usually easier to bring about than change of personality. However, even this is possible to the degree that obstacles to development are reduced or removed so that the patient is less anxious and more able to cope successfully with the crisis of growing up.

Enuresis

Occasionally enuresis of early childhood persists into adolescence. Some children have a smaller functional bladder size and a lesser capacity to hold urine for longer periods of time, or have learned the habit of urinating frequently during the daytime and during the night, with occasional incontinence in sleep. But even in these patients psychogenic factors are often manifest, either as influences which trigger the mechanism, or appear as reactive shame, disparagement of self and guilt. Stress experiences, such as school tests, upset adolescents as they do younger children and may cause them to wet themselves. Their embarrassment makes them shun contacts with peers.

The adolescent who returns to enuresis usually is one who is anxious and worried during his waking periods and whose sleep is disturbed by dreams of an aggressive or erotic nature. To some the enuresis is as pleasurable as an orgasm. When this occurs, children may not be highly motivated to give up the trait. On the other hand, the discomfort of a wet bed as well as the shame may act to overcome the difficulties for some individuals or cause them to seek help.

In attempting a cure, the explained use of a non-painful electric gadget to awaken the child by stimulation at the time of wetting has been successful. The use of the instrument, voluntarily applied, does not frighten the adolescent as it does younger children, but it does not remove any underlying psychologic difficulty.

Encopresis and Fecal Soiling

Like the pre-school child, the adolescent (particularly females) may build up fantasies about defecation and stools. Some liken having a bowel movement to delivering a baby, and endow feces with human characteristics. Although the retention of stool to the point of soiling is present in boys as well as in girls in adolescence, it is more common in the latter and endowed with a different kind of fantasy. The boy does not think so much of having a baby while he is having a bowel movement, but does humanize the stool and has thoughts of aggression toward its representation as he passes the feces into the toilet. Both sexes enjoy defecation and retain feces in order to prolong the act, because it has erotic-like sensations attached to it. This leads to an accumulation of feces much as in the pre-school child who holds back, causing involuntary soiling and paradoxical diarrhea (See p. 52). Some adolescents not only retain their stools in the bowel, but collect them after defecation. Where there is incontinence, the underwear may be saved instead of being laundered. Such individuals cannot explain the reasons for collecting the stools or their dirty underwear. Despite their shame at facing the parents who raise the question, they tend to continue the habit. Often this behavior is associated with other neurotic traits which indicate that psychiatric treatment should always be considered.

The problem is usually not brought to the pediatrician by the adolescent, but by his parents. It is understandable that they should urge the youth to stop hiding his clothing and insist that he launder his own underwear, but neither admonitions nor ridicule are effective as a cure. In this matter as in others involving highly charged feelings, it is difficult for parents and adolescents to discuss the behavior objectively and critically. For that reason the problem invariably is brought to a professional person, and the non-psychiatric physician is usually consulted first. The physician mistakenly is inclined to deal with the stool problem specifically as one of constipation, suggests stool softeners and the practice of going to the toilet regularly each day. Obviously, the child who is wilfully or unconsciously withholding stool will not be motivated to defecate regularly even if the stools are softer. Since stool accumulation is rarely as extreme to the point of chronic enlargement of the colon as in the pre-school period, it is not as imperative for the physician to focus on changing the character of the stool.

The doctor may be very helpful to the adolescent in providing an avenue for discussion, even though the problem may not respond directly. Through an accepting and reassuring experience with a respected physician the teenager is often enabled to give up his infantile habits and fears, improve his self-esteem and gain confidence in the growing up process with all its complexities. Just being understood is in itself a powerful and sustaining tonic for the adolescent.

Many young people sooner or later give up the habit of retaining stool, stop having fantasies about the feces and no longer soil. In girls who become pregnant there may be a resumption of the birth fantasy when they are constipated. For boys and girls who continue for several months without changing their habits of defecation, and who continue to be incontinent or have a paradoxical diarrhea, psychologic assessment is indicated. This is usually done best by a psychiatrist because it involves skill in interviewing in depth and in interpreting the symptoms. The non-psychiatric physician rarely has the time or the skill to serve the patient this way.

Peer Relationships

Peer groups serve a variety of purposes in adolescence. Opportunity is presented to compare one's self with one's fellows, to test one's self against others; socialization experiences are provided. The adolescent who is insecure may find support and security in a group. The group experience helps provide distance from involvement with the family and is therefore a buffering influence upon conflicts between the teen-ager and his family. Anxiety about his changing feelings towards his parents, particularly his hostility towards them, may be somewhat assuaged when he hears that others feel as he does. Furthermore, group membership offers an opportunity effectively to commit acts which an adolescent cannot do alone. Since society offers few opportunities for adolescents as a group, they seek alternatives in peer group activities. These may benefit society or serve as anti-social protests.

The adolescent who cannot form close relationships with one or two peers or learn to fit into a group, or who is rejected by one, feels increasingly lonely, unhappy and isolated. He may withdraw as a neurotic defense, or he may join or organize other groups whose actions serve his angry and aggressive feelings. The pediatrician may be called upon to advise parents about helping a youth to become more acceptable to a group. Often he is asked to recommend organizations where adolescents may find safe and healthy companionships. Usually such assistance becomes more effective if the pediatrician's relationship with his adolescent patient is a positive and significant one that enables the teen-ager to identify with the physician's attitude toward associating with and participating in the activities of a peer group.

The adolescent who has not been successful in attaining the satisfying peer associations may complain of ill health. The physical symptoms of illness are his ticket of admission to the physician rather than his feelings of unhappiness and rejection. Delinquency *per se* is rarely a problem for which medical help is sought by parents. Part of the reason is that asocial, particularly delinquent behavior, is usually covered up by middle- and upper-class parents. The occasional stealing, lying, or community escapade, while troublesome, is viewed as "wild oats" or is reminiscent of a parent's own "normal" youth. Not infrequently parents unwittingly sanction behavior, although overtly condemning it, as they unconsciously act out their own needs vicariously through the child. If repeated, especially if it brings shame and disgrace, then parents often precipitously demand professional help and effective advice. However, a parent with high standards may early bring his anxiety to the physician.

If there is an ongoing relationship between the adolescent and doctor, this heightens the specificity of the medical assessment and the usefulness of the advice. For example, the parents of a 14-year-old girl sought the assistance of their pediatrician because of her excited interest in boys and her rebellious reactions toward the limits set on dating. It became clear in the interview that the child's mother was encouraging her daughter's interest in boys by warning her of the importance of marriage and the dread of becoming a spinster. The pediatrician referred the mother to a social worker for assistance in clarifying her relationship to her daughter in order that the mother would know more clearly how to guide herself in helping her daughter to grow up.

The physician's role is to view the behavior developmentally, attempt to understand its meaning, and interpret it to the parents. Often the symptoms are those of mid-adolescent rebellion against parents which requires patience and endurance on their part. Advocating certain changes in parental handling may be effective. Other recommendations effecting the milieu may be helpful such as away-from-home experiences including schooling. However, sending an adolescent to a boarding school may fail because it may be inappropriate for a specific individual or because it may be viewed as punishment by exile.

One new and increasingly disturbing pattern in medical practice relates to sexual delinquency. It may be wrong to consider much of the present-day sexual freedom as representing potential or real delinquency. On the other hand it does seem that many adolescents today in their sexual experimentation are going to extremes. The girl who becomes pregnant out of wedlock, and the boy and girl who are promiscuous in their sexuality, cause concern to parents and to teachers. They ask the physician for advice in helping all parties concerned. Frequently these children require psychiatric therapy, even residential treatment. Unfortunately, the latter is difficult to obtain.

As in the management of so many problems relating to children, the role of the parents in helping delinquent youths is primary. They need guidance, education, reassurance, support, and understanding which help them handle anxieties stemming from their own attitudes in child rearing. They may feel guilt-ridden from failures to either assume responsibility in appropriate measure or at the right time; a conflict in standards between parents themselves may have led to inconsistency and divisive management. The child becomes confused because he lacks an appropriate parent figure to emulate, or because his allegiances are divided.

The physician's role in the community includes attempts to develop more and better opportunities for constructive social experiences and resources for emotionally disturbed patients. Often these adolescents are judged delinquent, and require treatment away from home. Sometimes the physician may be a model with whom such youth can identify. They seek him out as a trusted, experienced, friendly adult who they believe can help. The physician will serve them best if he demonstrates the qualities attributed to him, does not attempt to moralize, and does not act as a parent meting out criticism or punishment.

The physician should listen with understanding and due regard for the real concerns of the adolescent so as to help him understand and direct his behavior. A physician sometimes effectively helps an individual by meeting with him as one in a group of adolescents where each may learn from listening to the others. The fact of being accepted in a group of peers may be beneficial. The physician as group leader represents society at large as well as a specific person of authority. (See Group Meetings, pages 186–192.)

The pediatrician must be clear about his own moral choices in order to not impose them on his patients. He also must be clear about the health values that are guidelines for advice about sexual behavior for adolescents. These health values are based, in our opinion, on the assumption that sexual intercourse is a desirable experience, one that becomes increasingly complex and satisfying when a man and woman are biologically, socially and emotionally mature enough to form an exclusive affectionate relationship which is expected to be permanent.

Pediatricians often find their adolescent patients from middle-class backgrounds troubled by the conviction that they are not as adequate as they are supposed to be if they do not engage in sexual intercourse as soon as they reach college. For example, an 18-year-old boy asked to see his pediatrician when he returned home for his Christmas vacation. It became clear that his uncle had told him he should become a man by having intercourse when he left home. He found class mates at his college with a similar burden. To his pediatrician he expressed the fear that there was something seriously wrong with him as he had been unable to sustain an erection with a prostitute. The pediatrician listened carefully and simply asked the young man why he thought he was ready to have intercourse. This led to a clarification of the boy's fear that he was a homosexual—not a man—if he did not have intercourse, especially since he was fearful of being teased about his lack of manliness. He was greatly relieved when he and the pediatrician agreed that he was forcing himself to engage in intercourse out of fear rather than on the basis of a mutually affectionate relationship between a man and woman capable of a permanent commitment.

Chapter 8

PEDIATRIC EVALUATION

Correct Identification of the Patient and the Problem

The pediatrician faced with the problem of serving a patient no matter what the disorder has three fundamental aims: to enhance normal development, to prevent mental and physical disorders and to restore the physical and emotional health of the patient. The accomplishment of these ends is the epitome of medical practice. In pursuit of the ideal, the physician uses certain traditional methods: history-taking, examinations, formulation of a diagnosis, prescription of a regimen and the prediction of the course of the problem or disorder.

Although the physician may not view it as such, this is actually a form of clinical investigation in the true sense of the word. Each visit with a physician is an experiment in which the practitioner is presented with a problem, accumulates data, makes hypotheses, and tests them by various therapeutic measures. The vital elements of his research include direct observation, collection and recording of evidence, assessment of data and verification of hypotheses.

In our practice which involves the behavior problems of parents and children we combine the traditional approaches with clinical research investigation. Some modifications are necessary because such practice usually involves consideration of the dynamics of family life.

We have found it advantageous to rephrase our tasks of evaluation and management as follows:

1. Correct identification of the patient and the problem. (To take a history)
2. Thorough collection of the evidence. (To continue the history and make examinations)
3. Accurate assessment of the data. (To differentiate, diagnose and predict)
4. Solution of the problem (to plan and participate in care and management).

Within each of these categories we seek answers to specific questions which will give the most comprehensive understanding, knowledge and validation to guide us to a solution which will be of meaningful help to

11

the patient. In this chapter the first three items and their key questions will be discussed in detail. The fourth, dealing specifically with solution and management of the problem, will follow in Chapter 9.

The Preliminaries

Setting the Appointment

The helping process begins with the first contact between the person seeking help, and the physician or his representatives, usually a telephone receptionist or office nurse. The way she handles the call can aid to establish a suitable and accepting rapport with the parent. By sensing the tone of the request, such as hesitancy, urgency or hostility, the response should be helpfully geared to initiate a constructive atmosphere in the forthcoming appointment. The time and place for the interview appointment should foster ease of communication for a troubled person and a busy physician.

The giving of an appointment sets up anticipation in the parent and child; there are feelings of relief mixed with apprehension in both. The physician too is not immune from emotional involvement, although he may not be aware of such feelings unless they are strongly negative, as when he is uncomfortable and frustrated in facing behavior problems, or angry at a parent and disapproving of a child. The physician who enjoys his role takes a matter-of-fact pleasure in human interaction. The joy of practice comes from the view that the human organism, physically, emotionally and developmentally, is a perpetual challenge to his own knowledge, abilities and humanity. The secret of his success often lies in his own feelings and attitudes, as well as those of the patient.

Structuring the Appointment

There is benefit when the meeting time and place is structured. The giving of an appointment implies that there will be no hurried consultation, no curbstone advising like the kind some patients try to get at a cocktail party. The patient (and for our purpose, this is usually the parent-child couple) is told the length of time available at the beginning of the interview. From the physician's viewpoint this is necessary in realistic terms of his schedule. For the informant it is beneficial to know in advance how much time is at his disposal to say what he thinks is important.

However, the way that this is handled is all-important to the success of the interview. Consider for a moment the effect on an anxious and distraught individual when told by the physician "we have 30 minutes to discuss this matter." At the very least a pressured atmosphere results, if not resentment and hostility. On the other hand the remark that "I've allowed ample time of 30 minutes because I want the opportunity for a full discussion" will both set a time limit and convey the physician's interest and concern.

Hopefully a fixed period may minimize rambling talk and verbose reporting. But if the informant tends to ramble and repeat, or if his account seems verbose, this in itself is significant. It is especially a sign of apprehension, poor ability in expression, or even a testing out of the physician. The so-called "irrelevant talk" may have important meaning although the physician is not yet able to assess its relevance. The order in which the informant presents material may also be a clue to its importance.

If time is indeed running out, and if the issue remains totally obscure, a few specifically directed questions may force the informant to focus on basic questions. These may include asking "What do you think is the main problem?" or "How do you think I may help?" The patient will be more secure when the interview is structured around *his* chief presenting complaint, and the issues are at least "put on the table." Even if the physician knows that there are other underlying problem areas he must be wary of tackling too much on this first exposure.

Sometimes both parents are involved in the first or later interviews. This is all to the good. The physician has the opportunity to note the interaction between the parents, their individual interpretations and viewpoints of the complaint, their approaches to it. This can add immediate dimensions of understanding to the perceptive physician.

Since the first meeting involves talking at length about many things which may be pertinent or seem irrelevant, a longer time is alloted for this interview. It should vary from 30 to 60 minutes depending on the schedule of the doctor and his threshold of fatigue and patience. Contacts with the physician may be limited to one meeting, or there may be more over a period of months when he provides long-term care either as the single therapist, or as a member of a group of professional workers. His role in the latter arrangement may be that of a leader and primary supervisor, or as a less involved consultant. Whether short term or long, the essence of the helping process lies in the relationship of the persons involved, particularly that of physician to patient.

The Interview—Communication is the Key

Communication with the Parents

A good history gives the diagnosis. With this in mind each physician develops his own unique habits and techniques of carrying on an interview. He recognizes that different people require different approaches and styles of interviewing. Since what transpires depends on the success of communication, something special is demanded of the physician as well as the patient. Each must demonstrate good faith. Both must use words and concepts which are heard and clearly understood by the other; each must feel the undertones of what is being said and be receptive of the message.

The patient's interpretation of what the doctor has said is a good indication of whether the communication has been effective. Mutual understanding is a prerequisite in helping the patient, as well as the doctor's sincerity, friendliness, tact and concern. These attitudes are transmitted by the physician in various ways and in accordance with his own style, but they should be initiated at the first interview and remain an objective goal in all subsequent contact. If either party is too impatient, too lacking in confidence, too charged with feelings of anger or dislike, he will reject what the other says. Communication will be impaired.

A main obstacle to straightforward communication is the feeling of reticence and anxiety which leads the informant to talk about seemingly irrelevant and disassociated matters. A mother who is in an agony of fear that her son's pain in the leg may turn out to be leukemia may be unable to voice directly such a devastating concern. Instead she may ramble on about "growing pains," a respiratory infection, or lack of physical activity. Finally, in this circuitous route the physician may learn the genesis of the problem if he is not impatient; namely that a friend's son with an unexplained pain in the leg did develop leukemia.

Emotional blocking may be so severe that it paralyzes the informant's ability to come to grips with the problem. Out of need, people wear many masks. This should not disarm the physician. He should be aware that intense anxiety, deep hostility or overpowering guilt may well parade as nonchalance, flippancy or reserve. Sometimes physical symptoms such as flushed face, dry mouth or tremulous hands betray the true state of emotional feeling.

Some persons try to hide their apprehension by aggressively lashing out with complaints and demands for remedies which "cure" speedily. Not every parent who comes to a physician with a behavior problem wants help, despite such implication. The parent may have been sent by a school teacher and resents the concern as an intrusion in the family's personal affairs. In such instances she comes with a chip on her shoulder, mostly to complain against the teacher and to find support for her position from the physician.

It is not easy for the physician to remember that these feelings and attitudes are usually unconscious, rather than deliberate attempts to distort or make his work difficult. The doctor who listens "in depth" can discover some main thread of information which answers the questions he has put to himself, "What is she *really* talking about?" "*Who* has the problem?"

Sometimes there is deliberate falsification of a concern in order to permit the airing of a deeper and more basic one. It involves a "testing out" of the doctor, to prove himself so to speak, before the more painful concern is broached. An example of this was the middle-aged woman who brought her 11-year-old daughter to the clinic because of "repeated colds." The girl did not appear sick, had no complaint herself, and felt that her mother was unnecessarily worried about the three or four respiratory infections which she had each year.

The history as given was extremely diffuse. Attempts to clarify it were frustrating. However, 5 minutes before the end of the allotted time the mother suddenly poured out a series of family tragedies and realized that her real reason for coming was to talk about her husband who was a pyro-maniac. She felt the need to report him to someone, but had not had the courage to take the matter to the police. The "frequency of colds" was her ticket of admission to the physician. It was unwittingly chosen because she believed it would qualify her for an interview with him. Furthermore, talking to a physician about "a family problem" was less forbidding and safer than talking with the police about her husband's crimes.

A parent who feels guilty may also falsify her story. She may, for example, withhold facts about contacts with other physicians. Or she may refer to them but distort the advice she had received. Checking the mother's history (with her permission) with the other physicians, usually clarifies what transpired between them and what was the real regimen recommended.

History-taking is never a "one shot" proposition. It is a continuous dynamic process wherein data are accumulated beginning with the first interview and continuing throughout the physician-patient relationship. History-taking includes what is specifically communicated and what is observed and learned directly by the physician in office or home visits.

In pediatric history-taking, the situation is particularly complex because the "history" (biography) usually relates to a third person, with the mother serving as the clinical observer of her own child. Her observations therefore may be colored by emotion, ignorance or attempts to substantiate her own diagnosis. The physician is then forced to view the child first through the mother's eyes, and then decide on her accuracy. In making an objective assessment of the mother, it is invariable that he will bring in his subjective feelings as well.

Hence another obstacle to healthy physician-patient communication may be a conscious or unconscious feeling of antipathy between them. Just as a patient may be stressed by anxiety, hostility and guilt, so too the *doctor* may have similar emotional forces related to a particular patient. The presence of such feelings does not mean that the patient is necessarily of poor character, ignorant or lacking in positive motivation. Neither does it mean that the physician is inept or heartless. It is not unusual for a physician and a patient to overcome their antipathy as each is motivated by interest, or need to persevere and to continue the relationship. Feelings which are initially held may well be modified or changed. Barriers to communication are not uncommon and when they appear the physician must consider possible reasons and remove them early in the interview if at all possible.

If negative feelings should persist in the physician or in the patient, the severity of the problem and its need may make further interviews necessary despite the incompatibility. Sometimes there is no other community resource available to the person with the problem other than the physician. Therefore despite the existing limitations of rapport the doctor may be able to be of assistance. This in itself can change the tone of the relationship to one of greater reciprocity and cordiality.

But there are occasions when the physician must terminate contact with a patient with whom he feels he absolutely cannot work. If he rids himself of such a patient, labelling him ignorant, uncooperative or neurotic, it may serve the physician's own emotions, but it does not help the child or the parent. A frank but friendly suggestion to terminate because it is in the best interest of the patient would be advisable. Terminating on this basis may actually benefit a patient by providing opportunity for a new beginning with another physician, wherein there might be more effective communication and resolution of the problem.

To assure the kind of interview and communication which will lead to constructive resolution of the patient's problem the physician cannot be falsely reassuring or glib with superficial advising. Nor should he relate over-personally or over-identify to the point where his usefulness as an objective and qualified third party is diminished. The physician manages well if he listens carefully, clarifies the problem for the patient and himself, creates confidence and trust, feels friendliness, interest and concern for the patient.

Communication with the Child

Although the parent is usually the dominant informant and the one who begins the relationship with the physician, communication with the child is equally essential. In the instance of an infant or young child the parent will usually be the only one dealt with in the interview, but it will still be necessary to have contact with the child for independent observation and assessment. The manner of interview with the child is of course dependent on his age. An adolescent may seek help himself and be the primary informant with little involvement of his parents, especially the adolescent who is attempting to be independent of them.

There is always merit in listening to a child because it involves him actively in the management of his own problems. Some of the problems of communication with parents may be avoided when the child is of an age when he has the intelligence and the willingness to give his own story.

Talk with children must be treated with the same degree of confidentiality as are the comments by the parents. The physician's approach must convey respect for the child and his feelings, without criticism or disapproval. He should put the child at ease by a lead-in question concerning the child's feeling about coming to the doctor, or even a direct question as to why *he* thinks he was brought. This may be followed with a general remark about the apprehensions that most children feel in coming to the doctor. And he might add that all he plans to do is listen to anything the child would like to talk about.

Children may not be able accurately to reveal facts about themselves for the same reasons which hinder adults; apprehension, ignorance and even unawareness that "a problem" exists. Many children are puzzled about the reasons for coming to a doctor. They may even have been brought under false pretenses, as "for a checkup." Not only fairness but therapeutic success demands that a child know the true facts early in his contact with the physician. The child's age, cooperation and level of intelligence are all factors in how the doctor proceeds. In some instances his approach can be direct, in others quite indirect. He should respond to the child's clues, using each of them as a stepping stone to further the communication. It is of paramount importance that the physician's interview techniques be flexible and that he be sensitive to the child's feelings.

By his friendliness and by his words which honestly describe what he is doing the doctor reassures a child. He carries the interview forward not by relentless questioning and probing, but as "you care to tell about things which interest both of us." It is natural for the child to test the truth of the physician's statements, to hold back, or be unable to think about highly charged material until he trusts him. But children develop their feelings about their doctor from earliest years, so that rapport is easily re-established, even when the visit is for a reason not involving physical illness primarily.

Small children are understandably imprecise about their complaints and their life histories. Nevertheless, even children of 4 and 5 years of age often can speak meaningfully about their symptoms, whereas their mothers may present only vague remarks about them. The technique of interviewing a child is different when he is young and may entail playing with him rather than relying on direct conversation (See Chapter 9, Play Activity).

Detecting the Meaning of Behavior

The meaning of the behavior (the "problem") may be unclear to those who come to the doctor, as well as to the doctor himself. A major task of the physician is to try to determine its meaning; to give some interpretation to the patient so that with insight he may be helped (See Chapter 9, Therapeutic Management, p. 177). Unless he can successfully do so the physician fails the patient by treating only the symptom, as by prescribing drugs alone in an extreme instance. This is akin to prescribing a sedative and analgesic drugs for abdominal pain without attempting to determine its meaning.

The meaning of a behavioral trait is hard to determine for a number of reasons. The history may be vague or distorted as described before. The problem of the child may be largely symptomatic of parental difficulties. The child not only may be a projection of these difficulties, but may be used as a foil for them. But even when the child "is the patient," his behavior may mask a psychologic conflict, just as when pain masks physical illness.

The reason for this is that much of behavior is unconsciously determined. It is a defense mechanism of the child in that it brings some gain, even though it may be painful and abhorrent to both child and parents. In the clinical entities described in this book we have emphasized the psychologic mechanisms of symptom formation and the processes of restitution. These are not always apparent in an interview because they are not clearly overt.

The physician is tempted to look deeper when he fails to understand the child's behavior. There is some danger in this which the patient apprehends. He shows it by his facial expression, his manner of speech and by the way he backs away from a "hot" area. When a doctor inadvertently touches such a particularly painful area, great harm will not invariably follow if he recognizes the signs and retreats. For example, the topic of sex is still taboo for some, and may even be as difficult for the physician to face. The physician should learn how to cope with his feelings, uncertainty or ignorance, if he hopes to help the patient. Until then he will best avoid discussion about it. If the evidence suggests that the item is too complex or too threatening to be explored, referral to someone more expert is indicated.

Not all emotional conflicts are unconscious. Many are at a conscious and preconscious level which makes them more readily accessible and amenable to treatment. Many patients with psychosomatic disorders are aware of the stresses in their lives and of the emotional tensions which are the sources of their symptoms. The patient's difficulty is not so much in his inability nor unwillingness to recognize his emotions and so dissipate pathologic tension, but rather in his inability to talk about his feelings and share them with a physician.

Whether the patient be a parent or child, inability to express his conscious feelings should be recognized by the physician whose role then is to help him unburden his grievances or personal worries through discussion. In the case of the younger child, if he is not mature enough for that, acting out the problem in play will serve as well as communicating by talk. In the case of the adolescent or the adult the physician's technique must be sufficiently sophisticated to open the door to communication. He may lead in with a question about a previous remark of the patient; or he may comment that he noted a hesitancy when such and such was mentioned, or he may initially discuss a more neutral subject.

While a patient will remain vulnerable and the tension-producing experiences may continue, nevertheless in the release of pent-up feelings there may be a reduction of the pressure that keeps the behavior problem going. This in itself may reduce the amount of suffering and the degree of symptomatology. Periodic release of feelings gives encouragement to a patient and this in turn may diminish the feelings of stress.

One key in interviewing lies in the physician's attentive listening rather than aggressive questioning. Because emotionally traumatic material is painful to the persons involved, it is unlikely to emerge as long as the informant controls the flow of talk. In this regard, mention should be made that flagrant omissions of important topics, or silences, are just as significant as repetitious and verbose speech or provocative statements.

Invariably in listening to an informant, the physician becomes aware of areas which are tender and painful to the speaker. The physician then judiciously redirects the trend of talk. This is analogous to an abdominal palpation when the patient winces and the doctor instinctively takes note of his reaction but does not continue probing lest it stimulate the pathologic condition. The purpose is not to bottle up the informant or to avoid issues entirely because they are painful, but rather to postpone discussion of them until there is therapeutic benefit to be derived. The interview cannot hope to accomplish radical emotional surgery, only to open up the areas of illness to both doctor and patient. The patient is not only helped over the stressful period, but may be prevented from becoming more anxious and developing a panic. Deeper exploration can ensue when the patient returns for another appointment. Physicians learn to recognize danger signals and how to cope with patients from trial-and-error experience. Such greater sensitivity and earlier recognition brings self-confidence in management.

A useful rule to follow then is not to explore indiscriminately or without constraint, not to uncover material which is too threatening at the time so that it cannot be handled beneficially by the patient.

It is remarkable how much help may be given a disturbed patient, by hearing him out without trying to analyze his psyche. By his traditional authority, the physician still holds a unique position of trust. With that awareness the patient comes prepared to speak in confidence, to ventilate his feelings and attitudes because he feels it is safe to do so. This in itself is highly therapeutic.

Giving a second appointment, soon after the first, is often beneficial. It may help the informant clarify issues, bring in more accurate information, and especially return to topics which previously were painful, avoided, or described in a way which on further reflection seemed inaccurate or unwise. In talking a second time to the physician, feelings of guilt may force a restatement of the topic, as when a poor marital relationship which was previously exposed so critically is now minimized.

Often a physician wonders if he has missed a clue by not sufficiently recognizing a remark of a patient, because he was insensitive to it or timid about exploring it. It will comfort him to know that a patient tends to return to topics which consciously or unconsciously are particularly meaningful to him and his problem. Thus the physician has more than one opportunity to hear and constructively use the material in diagnosis and treatment.

Thorough Collection of the Evidence

The Complaint

In the traditional sense this involves *history-taking, recording information,* and *arranging the data in chronological terms.* This is to show the temporal events of the patient's biography in conjuction with its meaningful relationships to family and community. The physician attempts to determine facts about the *present* difficulty, *what* the problem is, *who* is concerned, what the *circumstances of coming* are, as well as the *nature of the people* with whom he is becoming involved.

But history-taking is not only to collect information, but also to bring about an emotional release during the recital. It is in such an indirect manner that therapy actually begins. Thus despite the need to acquire vital background information, the physician must not be so hurried or become so engrossed in questioning that he leaves no time to discuss the *actual* complaint or immediate problem which brought the patient in the first place. Some physicians request a brief written statement about the problem preliminary to the interview. This may include some historic data or might even consist of answers to specific questions in questionnaire form. The practicality of this depends, of course, on the interest of the parents, their ability and willingness to take the time. Such information may suggest the nature of the problem, but it often is scanty or inaccurate. (See Computerized History-Taking, page 158.)

Ideally the interview should entail spontaneous talking by the informant about the specific complaint, description of the behavior, identification of the time and circumstances under which it arose and what followed. Invariably some comments about his feelings and attitudes along with specific facts and general information will be included.

The physician may interject a question now and then, to clarify a fact or to emphasize a point, which helps the informant get some insight into the nature of the problem and its genesis; a carefully directed and well-timed question also has therapeutic potential. For example, "I can see that as a good mother you tried to protect your child. Do you believe you over-protected her?"

The Past and Family Histories

The account of the present illness leads naturally to a consideration of the *events which preceded the onset,* especially identification of the *precipitating agents,* and description of those *measures taken to modify the disorder.* The family history then follows. This should provide not only facts about ages and health of parents, especially *genetic backgrounds* when certain inherited disorders are suspected, but also *description of the psychologic relationships* of the family members. Since most behavior problems are associated primarily with defects in parent-child relationships, main issues to be faced are those involving parental attitudes and feelings which reflect conflicts with children.

Parenthetically, if circumstances should arise where a visit to the home takes place, this can be an excellent opportunity to acquire information. The parental behavior under such conditions, the atmosphere of the home, the interaction of parents-child, all provide dimensions of observation and understanding most valuable to the perceptive physician.

A discussion of *child-rearing practices* with parents invariably leads to talk about their needs, hopes, expectations, disappointments and failures. Recitation of these highly personal and emotionally charged areas not only gives the doctor some insight into the origin of the behavior problem, but may even give the parent some insight into his role in its development. For example, a parent may recognize her over-concern, overindulgence, neglect or lack of consistency as she describes her way of dealing with her child.

On the other hand parents are also quick to react in defense of their own attitudes and practices, and look to the child for his deficiencies. At this point in the history-taking, the physician should inquire further about the *developmental history of the child* and obtain a *description of his personality,* its strengths and vulnerability to stress, and patterns of reacting behaviorally. The parent already will have talked about some of this in describing the behavior problem and its effect on the child, the parent and others. A detailed review of his personality, behavior and development helps one to understand the normality or deviancy of the child's behavior by comparing him with his peers (See Developmental Schema Charts). For example, some children are excessively fearful, overly shy and reserved. These traits may denote a child's lowered threshold to emotional stress and his difficulty in coping with it, or they may have other meaning.

The physician may be helped to see temporal relationships between events by constructing a *life chart* of the patient. The chart is arranged in four columns wherein each fact is noted with regard to the time of its occurrence. The first column contains the dates and ages of the child beginning with birth; the second, pertinent facts of physical development and somatic illnesses; the third, changes in living conditions, school and work, illnesses and deaths in the family; and fourth, the personality reactions which have occurred at various times. In effect, this is a summary of the "medical history." (It may be used in discussing diagnosis and treatment with a parent because it facilitates the conceptualization of the formation of a behavior problem.)

In looking for temporal relationships between stressful events in a patient's life and the occurrence of symptoms, the physician should not only determine major single events, such as loss of parents or separation from them by hospitalization, but even those which are considered minor by the doctor's standards. For the *patient* they may be extremely meaningful. The number of times an event occurs, the consistency with which symptoms appear, and the emotional display and attitudes of parent and child at the time of the event are all noteworthy. For example, sleeplessness after every new experience indicates a primary reaction pattern of significance. No display of emotions, or no report of their display, indicates repression or denial of the psychologic significance of an event. The physician should also record what measures relieve symptoms; the familiar therapeutic test.

It will also be helpful if the degree of emotional reaction to an event is determined. People do not become *equally* angry even though their response in general may be similar to the same event. Furthermore, people handle their feelings differently depending on the meaning of an event for each of them. Temporal relationships are not always recognized because of the latent period between stress and symptom; the so-called "sleeper effect" is notorious in children's behavior. Reactions to events do not always manifest themselves in a few hours, days or weeks; it may take many months for a reaction to appear, or to be in a form recognized by the patient or parent.

Computerized History-Taking

It is inevitable that computers will be used increasingly in the future for collecting and processing information about patients in order to help make a diagnosis and plan treatment. Already there are experiments in the direction of using questionnaires which patients fill out either before they visit their physician, or in his office while viewing questions on a TV screen. The questionnaire is arranged according to age and topic. Parents are asked to check items on the child's behavior such as whether he wets the bed, has bad dreams, sleeps restlessly, sucks his thumb, stammers, is high-strung and many others. They are also asked about their attitudes towards the children, towards their spouse and about their child-rearing practices. Questionnaires differ as to whether the respondent is merely to check the presence or absence of an item, while others graduate the responses from "Always" to "Never" in order to give some quantitative weight to the reply.

The aims of such mechanized approaches are laudable. They are to save the time of a busy practitioner, and to increase the accuracy of history-taking, particularly about events which may have been forgotten or which are so highly tinged with emotion that they cannot be explored accurately in the presence of the physician. Further, the patient has the opportunity to describe his symptoms at greater length and in more detail than a doctor's time permits.

In actuality questionnaire history-taking is not highly respected today. Often the respondents have filled out the questionnaires hurriedly, without much reflection. The result is that frequently they are incomplete and more inaccurate than histories obtained vis-a-vis in an interview.

Another disadvantage to the use of any device for collecting data and processing them arises from the fact that the instrument is not able to pick up the nuance of feeling which an intuitive and perceptive physician is able to do when he interviews a patient. Accordingly clues are missed which help identify what is relevant, pertinent and provocative.

In using the questionnaires as screening devices in diagnosis, false-positive and false-negative responses have been obtained, as in many laboratory tests. This is accounted for in part by the fact that in the field of behavior, unlike that of physical disorders, it is impossible to classify data clearly into psychologic entities, or diseases, or even to group symptoms meaningfully into terms of clinical significance. We have already stressed this in pointing out the difficulty a physician has in accurately assessing relevant data and arriving at a diagnosis of "what is normal" or what is abnormal in the behavior of a particular child even when in direct confrontation with the patient.

Finally, there is the further risk of impersonalization as when an instrument or device affords the physician opportunity to avoid personal contact with the patient. A computer can never replace a human being in a relationship, and while some physicians would like to be so replaced with some patients, no patient ever chooses it.

It may be assumed that despite the faults of the questionnaire there will be continued efforts to improve the mechanical collection and processing of historic data about patients. This being so, it is hoped that the time saved will permit the physician to give more of himself not only as someone to program the computer, but more to listen to the patient and talk with him in ways which are psychotherapeutic. It would be a tragedy if the physician found it impossible to give personally in helping the patient and relied on artificial aids.

Books and pamphlets on human behavior, relationships, physical health, and child-rearing, undoubtedly have educational value to some parents, yet none of these materials significantly relieve the anxiety, or change these attitudes of a parent and a patient, which have been developed as habits over a long period of time. There is still no substitute for a supportive person-to-person relationship between physician-patient.

The Physical Examination

For the physician to acquire evidence which is as complete as possible, he must go beyond history-taking. This usually means that the child is to be examined by the doctor, and occasionally by others such as a psychologist. Even when a physician believes that a behavior disorder is purely psychologic, he should consider the advantages and contra-indications of performing a physical examination. Obviously where the differential diagnosis is between physical and psychologic illness, and even when the former may be secondary to the latter, a thorough and competently done examination supplies information and reassures both physician and parent.

Both the timing of a physical examination and the manner in which it is performed are important. In our practice we have frequently postponed a physical examination until after we have had at least one lengthy interview with the parent, and a chance to talk with the child and observe him. This is particularly important in terms of the need to establish a friendly and trusting rapport with the child. If one examines the child in a way which was painful or embarrassing to him, rapport is not easily re-established and may never be. An opportunity for history-taking from the child presents itself during examination. By having him then give an account of his symptoms, life experiences and relationships with other persons, he may also be diverted from apprehension about the examination and resistance to it.

Unlike psychiatrists, we have not found the physical examination by the physician doing the complete work-up to be a deterrent to psychologic helping. However, when it is of benefit to a patient not to examine, as with a female when a gynecologic examination is indicated, we have referred such a patient to a competent and psychologically minded colleague. The reason for the referral is explained to the child along with a description of the examination.

Once a physical examination has been performed, there is no need to repeat it solely to reassure a parent. Repeated examinations may have the opposite effect, especially when the physician has already assured him that no physical illness exists. It may actually make a parent distrustful of the physician and dubious about his competency. Sometimes a parent suspects the physician's intent as selfish and money-oriented. Furthermore a complaint may become chronic if a physician reinforces it by requesting follow-up visits and re-examinations.

The extent of other examinations particularly neurologic, psychologic, developmental and electroencephalogram depend upon the physician's experience, judgment, and ability to deal with problems that are not traditionally pediatric. Laboratory and other investigations are not substitutes for careful history-taking, interviewing, or a physical examination competently done by a pediatrician.

Psychologic Testing

Some parents feel that their children have not been thoroughly studied unless examined by a physician and given mental tests. Others view psychologic testing with suspicion. In this event the physician is doubly required to explain the purposes and value of these laboratory aids which are extremely helpful in complementing a pediatric examination.

Although intelligence testing in a broad sense is part of every pediatric examination, clinical judgment of the physician about the child's intelligence is often fallacious. This may be so despite careful evaluation of the history provided by the mother and observation of the child and his responses to questions. It is particularly true when the patient is an infant and a young child.

Too frequently the physician errs on the side of not considering seriously the possibility of mental retardation. Many physicians still find it difficult to raise forthrightly the possibility with a parent that his child may be functioning at a retarded level. It is still common today for a parent to be told "not to worry about slowness of development because he will catch up sooner or later." This may be true but it must not be a snap, superficial or baseless reassurance.

In addition to tests of intelligence there are varieties of objective tests of personality, emotional development, and of parental attitudes. An excellent detailed description of most of these tests and the application of testing data may be found in a report of the Committee on the Handicapped Child published by the American Academy of Pediatrics in 1962. The following list of frequently used psychologic tests strikes a balance between those which are most useful and those most likely to be referred to in reports that come into the hands of a pediatrician. All the tests chosen rank high in frequency of use in hospitals, clinics and institutions.

Intelligence Tests. Stanford-Binet Intelligence Test (Forms L and M). This is a general test of intelligence standardized for 2 to 18 years of age. At the lower age levels it includes perceptual-motor tasks as well as verbal tasks but at higher age levels it becomes increasingly a verbal test of general intelligence. This intelligence test is highly recommended for use with normal children over 2 and under 18 years of age. It is also a good choice for use with moderately or severely retarded children who are functioning above a mental age of 2 years. This test is also to be recommended with cerebral palsied, blind and deaf children even though it requires modifications.

Wechsler Intelligence Scale for Children (frequently referred to as the WISC). This is a general test of intelligence standardized for 5 through 15 years of age. The test includes a Verbal and Performance Scale and permits a ready contrast between verbal and perceptual-motor aspects of intelligence. Within the scale there are six sub-tests which permit the measurement of intellectual functioning as arithmetical ability, general information and skills of perceptual organization. This test is less helpful for average or below average children under the age of 8 years. The adult forms of this test, the Wechsler Adult Intelligence Scale (WAIS) and the Wechsler-Bellevue are quite commonly used with older adolescents.

Draw-A-Man (Goodenough Test). This is a simple, non-verbal test of intelligence which requires a child to make a pencil and paper drawing of a man. The drawing is scored on the basis of the number of anatomic parts, items of clothing and motor co-ordination displayed in the drawing. Age norms are available from 3 to 13 years of age. The test results correlate fairly well with I.Q.'s derived from the Stanford-Binet, especially between the ages of 4 and 10 years. It should never be used by itself, but only as a supplement to one of the standard I.Q. scales where it can serve to modify or support the impression gained from a fuller testing of intellectual abilities.

Developmental Tests. The Gesell Developmental Schedules. These are scaled for the measurement of development from the first weeks of life through 5 years of age. The arrangement of the test items permits separate assessments of the following developmental areas: motor development, adaptive behavior, language development and personal-social behavior. As compared with the intelligence tests mentioned above, or even with other infant scales, the reporting of the standardization of this test is lacking in detail and clarity. Nevertheless it is a good tool for estimating the over-all development of the child under 2 years, or for estimating the development of the older but severely retarded or neurologically handicapped pre-schooler. (See Prediction of Development, pages 169–176.)

Cattell Infant Intelligence Scale. This is a downward extension of the Stanford-Binet Intelligence Scale. It yields mental age scores and I.Q.'s applicable to the child from 3 to 30 months of age. It seems better standardized than the Gesell developmental test but the word intelligence in its title may be misleading. In the use of the word in regard to the school child, most of us consider intelligence to involve complex processes of mentation. The meaning of "intelligence" of a 3-month-old infant is still ill-defined.

Personality Tests. Rorschach. A test of apperception consisting of ten ink blots. In these ambiguous stimuli, the subject reports the various things that he sees. The responses are then analyzed from the viewpoint of the determinants in the contents of the responses. From an analysis of what is seen and how it is seen, the clinician attempts to infer the dynamics and structure of the personality. This is the most widely used and most thoroughly investigated projective technique. As a clinical tool, it lacks the well-grounded validity of intelligence testing. In the hands of a competent clinician, it is a valuable adjunct to the psychiatric interview and case history.

Thematic Apperception Test. Devised by Professor H. A. Murray of Harvard, it is a projective test in which the subject is instructed to make up stories about pictures which he is asked to look at. Each picture represents a scene suggestive of various kinds of interpersonal relationships and dramatic situations. The stories and descriptions of the pictures can be used to make inferences concerning the emotions, conflicts, drives, defenses and value systems of the storyteller. This test has many variants for use with school-age children. One which is particularly well-known is the Michigan Picture Test which unlike the Thematic Apperception Test are pictures of actual school situations. The Rorschach and TAT are good complementary tests, with the latter revealing more of the surface features.

Draw-A-Person Test. This is a derivation of the Goodenough Intelligence Test put to projective use. The subject is asked to draw a person and it is assumed that this drawing will permit one to draw conclusions about the subject's body image and his attitudes towards himself and his body.

Special Diagnostic Tests. Visual-Motor Gestalt Test. Also known as the *Bender,* it consists of nine geometrical designs which the subject is required to reproduce with paper and pencil. It is sensitive to the diagnosis of brain damage. It is assumed that it is especially suited to assess the type of perceptual-motor defect so often found in that condition.

The Merrill-Palmer Performance Scale. This is used in diagnosing cerebral palsy in children who have little speech.

12

The Vineland Social Maturity Scale which is an over-all measure of social maturity, competency and intelligence for special use with mentally retarded children. Information may be obtained from the parent or other informant if the child is unable to give it himself.

For the greatest value, such tests should be performed (like all laboratory tests) by specially trained and experienced persons. A physician usually has neither the time nor the competence to do them well. There is, however, a modified developmental appraisal test by Provence that can competently and routinely be performed by the physician (See Prediction of Mental Development, pages 172–174.)

Preparation of Parents and Child for Testing. The physician should prepare the child as well as the parent for psychologic testing by following these principles. Never lie to the child. Tell him truthfully in a general way the nature of the test, the number of visits that will be required, the reasons for it. It is fair to say that the tests are like games and that they should be enjoyable. They should *never* be likened to "tests in school," particularly for a child who may have a school phobia. The psychologist who will do the testing should be identified by name and described as a person who is interested in children; not a teacher, not a doctor, not a psychiatrist.

The parents should be told honestly the full aims, purposes, methods and procedures inherent in psychologic testing, including the possibility of a re-take should circumstances of the test be less than optimal. Permission from parents should always be obtained before psychologic testing. They should be reassured that the tests are not "playing games," but ways of attempting to objectively assess the intelligence of the child, the nature of his personality, clues about his problems and concerns. They should be advised that the pediatrician or the psychologist will interpret and fully discuss the results of the tests with them.

After testing, the psychologist will share his results with the pediatrician. There should not be undue focus on the I.Q. as a number or a measurement of intelligence which is too narrowly interpreted. Information to the parent should not be confusing, or in conflict with information which the tester has given the parent. If the parent requests a written report, it should be provided by the psychologist for the professional person designated by the parents. Information which a psychologist feels is confidential should not be given to the school or to persons other than the parents without their written permission. Ordinarily we do not give the report to parents since it may be misinterpreted.

If it is at all practical, the pediatrician should observe the psychologic testing of his patients in order to get a new concept of the child's behavior under testing circumstances. He will also be better able to use the psychologic evaluation after he has witnessed the testing. Sometimes testing is unsatisfactory because a child is physically sick, irritable, frightened, or because there is something in the relationship between tester and child which prevents the establishment of a good rapport. When this happens, time will be saved if the examination is postponed and attempted under more satisfactory circumstances.

Where a pediatrician practices in a group, the part-time services of a psychologist on a regular basis may prove profitable in many ways. For one, knowledgeable parents today take it for granted that psychologic services are more or less routinely part of good pediatric care. For another, it is easy to refer to a person who is in one's office and the physician finds it easier to communicate with him, to understand his method of working, and his way of interpreting the test results. On his part, the psychologist understands the interests of the pediatrician and is readily available for informal discussion about topics in general, or patients in particular. Such a psychologist may also serve as someone to do play therapy with children. (See page 206.)

Accurate Assessment of the Data: Appraising the Relevant Differential Diagnosis

The process of sifting the relevant from the unimportant begins with history-taking and continues through the physical examination. However, a more accurate review and systematic formulation is possible only when all reports are in mind. Differential diagnosis is a weighing of all evidence. If the evidence is viewed and considered in the presence of the parent and the child, it is educational and helpful to them as well. It leads the physician to an assessment of his own skills and interests, and a decision as to what his appropriate role should be.

One of the first questions facing the physician is whether something is really wrong with the child. Even though a child's behavior is unacceptable to an adult, nothing may be wrong in the sense of a developmental aberration or deviant behavior. It may be that he is acting in a healthy and normal fashion and that his behavior is appropriate for him at that time in his life and for his type of interpersonal relationships.

Gauging Normality

In reviewing behavior of the child and attitude of the parent, there are certain yardsticks which may help answer the question "What is normal?"

1. *The developmental phase of a child; the developmental phase of the parent;* the pertinence to what is expected at that time. There are

phase-specific anxieties and conflicts. For example, a child upon entering nursery school or kindergarten has some separation anxiety about leaving parents and becoming independent. Probably his mother shares these feelings. An adolescent is in conflict about his sexual role and shows anxiety with his peers. His parents are concerned about his adjustment. These are normal for child and parent at those times.

2. *The community mores, neighborhood expectations and general culture;* the demands of the child's milieu. For example, some children are considered pathologically hyperaggressive but in reality their behavior is normal, natural and even necessary for survival in the community where they live and the circumstances under which they are reared. Or overly-polite behavior may indicate lack of confidence, yet it may be a quality demanded in a special school or by particular parents who traditionally expect mannerliness in children.

3. *Elaborateness of behavior pattern;* is it exaggerated? For example, it may be normal in a 4 year old to bed wet but if it is accompanied by a compulsive leaving of the bed in order to sleep with a parent, it indicates something more. The child may be overly-anxious or the parent overly-protective in admitting the child to her bed as a health measure.

4. *Tenacity of a behavior pattern;* its history of persistence. Some traits come and go as normal defense mechanisms, or evidences of a child's attempts to cope with life. On the other hand, the disorder may persist over time or reappear frequently. For example, bedwetting which persists long beyond the pre-school age is symptomatic of chronic illness, mental or physical.

5. *Intensity and spread of the trait;* its pervasiveness. The "weepy" child may be one who is normally sensitive and shy. But he may also be one who takes each new and threatening experience with such sensitivity that he not only weeps, but also withdraws more and more from contacts with others to the point of psychotic isolation. Or, for example, temper tantrums may be mild outbursts of legitimate anger, but they may also become deep and ferocious outbursts which carry with them the connotation of self-injury or destruction of others.

6. *The temporal relationship of behavior and experience;* timetable of event and effect. Although much of behavior in later life stems from early life experiences, one needs to try to detect the duration of time between event and its effect. Behavior in response to something in the immediate past is more apt to be temporary and appropriate to the circumstances. But it is clinically more serious, other things being equal, when it represents a carry-over experience from early life, and especially when it is repeated often or persistently.

7. *Cluster of traits;* addenda of problems. In general a single behavior trait less often indicates a pathologic condition than a cluster or group, although this is not necessarily a clear-cut test of normality. For example,

delinquency embraces a cluster of traits including lying, stealing, and law breaking. But lying alone might simply indicate a realistic avoidance or evasion which harms no one. However, if the lying should become persistent and pervasive, it might be considered pre-delinquent, even though not overtly accompanied by stealing or aggressive anti-social acts.

8. *Response to therapeutic measures;* healthful resiliency. Some parents and children change their ways of behaving and reacting to stress with a small amount of professional help, especially reassurance, and with encouragement from peers or adults. We say they are resilient and have reserve powers for psychologic repair. It has been proved many times that behavior which is worrisome or deemed pathologic by somebody, responds surprisingly well after little or no treatment. This in itself is an affirmation of gauging normality.

When the diagnosis "normal" has been made, the job is to confirm this opinion in the minds of those persons who are concerned; to *convince* them to accept the diagnosis of normality. This entails dealing with their anxiety as well as with the practicalities of the situation. It is much more than simply telling them that "all is well."

The parent should be told why the evidence leads to a conclusion of normality; why the behavior is developmentally and physiologically acceptable. The pediatrician's evidence and interpretation should be meticulously spelled out to reinforce his position. If it appears that this is not enough, the pediatrician must then cope further with the core problem—the parent's undue concern and anxiety. There are many ways to do this, depending on the patient and the circumstances. In some cases the pediatrician may offer (but not insist upon) a repeat visit by the parent alone in about a month. This in itself may be so reassuring that it will be no surprise if the appointment is cancelled because the problem has diminished. In other cases the pediatrician may find it useful to refer the parent to others for counselling or therapy (See Paramedical Support, pp. 203–206).

When there is evidence to show that the child's behavior is deviant and inappropriate, the physician must also justify his diagnosis. This entails interpreting the evidence diagnostically, explaining its meaning and helping the parent to understand the genesis of the behavior. The parent may counter with his own diagnostic formulation. He should be listened to because this may be the time to determine finally what he really wants and expects, what he is ready to accept.

If a parent rejects a diagnosis, the physician should resist giving interpretations which the parent is not ready to accept. Mention was made earlier that behavior, however distressing it may be to a person, has special meaning and some gain for him. Parental over-concern may be a reaction to basic rejection of a child, and helps the parent deal with the child in a way which seems more acceptable and a "lesser evil" to those who judge. A child's abdominal pain, however worrisome to a parent, is a more acceptable reason for avoiding school than is an "irrational" fear. In each example, an interpretation of the psychodynamic mechanisms may add stress to the conflict as parent and child react to such insight with guilt. Affixing a psychologic label and explaining its mechanisms may give intellectual insight and temporary comfort but usually it does not remove the trait because the psychologic forces behind it remain unaffected. Interpreting parental overconcern as rejection does not make a parent accepting of a child; telling a child that he is sick to avoid going to school does not lift his phobia.

Prognosis

The parent wants to know the prognosis, with and without treatment. Prediction is even more hazardous in the practice of psychologic medicine than in the management of physical illness. The physician should not be trapped into making light of a behavior disorder in order to avoid a parent's dismay or criticism of lengthy and costly treatment which may be involved. Furthermore, the physician should make clear that cessation of a given symptom does not necessarily mean basic improvement or even real benefit.

It is not unusual for a trait to stop after one reassuring interview with a doctor, so powerful may be the effect of suggestion, the authority of his position or personality. For example, enuresis may be halted by a physician whose approach and rapport is such that "the magic" occurred. Even the knowledge that the interview would take place and that the problem would soon be in the doctor's lap might be enough to end the pressures—and the enuresis. While such a result is laudable in that it gives relief to those who are upset and proves that change can be brought about, basically the change may be over-valued and represent undue optimism. Significant changes in a patient's personality or in his life situation are needed to insure more durable gains.

A behavior disorder may return, with the same or with other symptoms. This discourages parents and children and is variously interpreted, usually with over-pessimism. The physician should also be prepared for the development of symptoms in other family members as the patient is released from his symptoms. This is so because the pathologic equilibrium maintained by the family group in relation to the patient's disorder now shifts. When the patient and his symptoms change, the group equilibrium is affected—new patterns of adjustment must be found.

Prognosis is dependent on many factors; especially chronicity of a disorder, the type and degree of illness, the remediability, and the efficacy of therapeutic management.

*Prediction of Mental Development**

Issues frequently arise today in pediatric practice which exercise the possibilities and limitations of predicting development. It is therefore appropriate and necessary to consider this question. Predicting the development of the child has certain parallels to the more familiar role of the physician in assessing disease, including its etiology, symptomatology, course, and specificity of therapeutic measures. In this the competent physician has already learned to acknowledge the biologic and social complexity of the individual patient, while using specific and empirical knowledge about disease.

Developmental prediction also depends on a firm knowledge of the biologic and social factors inherent in the individual young organism and the expected course within such a framework. However, it is a complex, multidimensional question, rather than a simple one. Predictions of development are reliable under certain conditions and unreliable in others. The pediatrician can and should be willing to make predictions in some cases and not in others. The availability of a child development specialist who understands not only the techniques of assessment, but its validity under the various applicable conditions, will be of assistance to him as will his other medical colleagues.

Generally, it is now accepted that inborn and experiential factors codetermine the development of the child, and that it occurs in a dynamic, unfolding process. This comes about through an interaction of inborn, maturing systems and the forces of the environment. In the process of maturation both somatic and mental innate factors are called successively into play, according to an inherent biologic timetable.

We are accustomed to considering innate constitutional factors in understanding the development of the body and its organ systems, but this concept is more inclusive than that. The infant's constitution also includes primitive forms of the mental equipment that serves perception, motility, thinking, memory and other abilities which help the individual gradually to perceive and deal with reality. It includes the psychic drives which have their own maturational phases. One of the infant's needs is for an environment in which all of these maturing systems, somatic and psychic, can be organized into functional units and integrated with other functions and systems at successively higher levels. The crucial role of adequate nurturing and of other experiential factors in influencing the child's development have been amply documented.

If an infant is developing well, we assume (*i.e.* predict) that he will continue to do so. For example, in respect to motor development, if the infant creeps and pulls to stand at the expected time, we assume that he will walk and run similarly normatively. If the pre-stages of speech

* Based largely on contributions of Dr. Sally Provence.

are present, *i.e.* the social vocalization, the ability to make vowel and consonant sounds and later to combine them, we assume that speech will develop normally. In making this prediction we are also assuming the influence of an environment in which at least the child's most important developmental needs are met.

It is obvious that the accuracy of predictions lies in the fact that most infants are born with the potential for adequate development, and that many are reared in acceptable environments. It also takes into account that the normal early phases of the maturational process reflecting normal structural and biochemical processes are likely to be followed by similarly normal processes later. This kind of prediction is based upon *probabilities.* However it is important to note that there are inborn disorders of development which become manifest not in early infancy but only later. We are also aware that probabilities help very little in the specific situation of a particular patient.

In many instances the validity of such probability predictions have not altogether stood the test, even with neonates who have the physical characteristics of mongolism, microcephaly, gargoylism, craniofacial dysostosis and many other defects recognizable at birth or in the earliest months of life. Assumptions about these children are obviously based upon accumulated knowledge about outcome in other children with similar traits. Hence the assumption that *all* children with these physical traits would be similarly affected. Yet as experience accumulates and as variations of the originally described picture become evident, we have to extend our conceptions and revise our predictions. Formerly children who were called mongolian idiots were assumed to be remarkably uniform in mental capacity and personality. Later they were shown to have a rather wide variation in the eventual level of intellectual ability.

Disturbances in amino acid, carbohydrate, endocrine, and pigment metabolisms are being continuously explored since biochemical genetics has provided an approach to understanding them. However, the very advances in these areas rule out firm answers about what can be predicted. Such answers are likely to be out of date before they are even disseminated. It is already recognized that there is no one predictable developmental outcome for infants with phenylketonuria, congenital hypothyroidism or galactosemia.

The examination of chromosomal material is another burgeoning field which may provide highly relevant predictive information. But its significance will not be adequately understood until children can be followed over a period of years. Hence long range predictions about the mental development of an individual child should be made only with the greatest caution in many of these disorders, and probably only after a period of observation during which sequential developmental assessments are done.

How then do we approach the problem of predicting development? Thus far the major and most reliable source has been derived mainly from the clinical developmental and psychologic tests. The predictive diagnosis of neurologic development in the first few years of life is possible because maturation in the fetus and infant proceeds in an orderly fashion following a neurophysiologic timetable. Using the Gesell Developmental Examination, or modifications developed by Knobloch, Provence, and others, the pediatrician has an instrument which may with accuracy detect signs of normal neuromuscular development, major and minor neuro-abnormality (brain damage) and mental deficiency. Much can be said from these tests about the functional integrity of the central nervous system and, in the absence of pathologic signs, it may be inferred that the infant has a reasonable chance of attaining normal or better than average intelligence.

However, in terms of clinically predicting future intelligence such tests have been a matter of controversy. The situations in which such predictions proved incorrect were as frequent as those in which they were correct. Developmental tests, like others the clinician uses, have significant values and limitations. In assessing their values the significant question, according to Provence, is not "do infant tests have predictive value?" but "under what conditions and in regard to what developmental disorders can the scores on infant tests be closely correlated with scores obtained on tests of intelligence at later ages?" Posed in this way the question can be examined more relevantly.

In general, it can be said that early and later scores on tests correlate most closely when a "non-correctable," recognizable inborn biologic defect is involved, such as mongolism or primary microcephaly. When a correctable or at least treatable disorder is involved such as phenylketonuria or cretinism, test scores may change markedly over time, depending upon the timing of treatment and extent to which correction of the metabolic or endocrine defect is possible.

It is also different when circumnatal insults to the central nervous system from such problems as hypoxia at birth or hemolytic disease of the newborn damage a brain which heretofore has developed normally. Even in the presence of damage, the child may be endowed with a strong thrust toward normal development. Obviously, outcome will be related to the extent and location of the damage. If the infant has motor tract involvement which is one of the common visible abnormalities, and one tries to predict future mental development from a test which contains many items dependent upon motor ability, such a prediction is a silly exercise. The experienced child development specialist will not expect that a D.Q. (development quotient) of 60 in such a child can be projected forward in time to an I.Q. (intelligence quotient) of 60 at age 5, 6, or 10 years.

The situation also differs when environmental conditions have resulted in the infant's experiencing deprivation or trauma such as often occur in institutional settings and in families in which parents are unable to nurture their children. There are many reports, both from clinical and research sources, of the detrimental effect on the child's development of such life experiences. A developmental test done during the early years and at a time when the child is still having such an experience, assesses his condition at that point in time and is one of the most valuable means of specifying the ways and the degree to which his development has been impeded.

Obviously the outcome for the child depends upon how his development can be facilitated through improving his situation by whatever methods are indicated. The beneficial effect of improved care which addresses itself to his deficits and to his ongoing developmental needs is often quite dramatic. Residual effects of severe or long term deprivation and of traumatic experiences are, however, often visible in the child's personality development, in his physical growth, and in the level and style of intellectual functioning. In respect to adverse environmental conditions, as well as in some of the inborn metabolic errors, it may require several years in an improved situation and serial assessments of progress to predict future development with some degree of confidence.

Provence has modified the Gesell Developmental Examination to serve as a simple and practical test for measuring an infant's psychologic status. This is an observation schema with the infant and his parents as subjects. It is easily performed because it includes most items which a pediatrician usually incorporates into his physical examination. Fundamental to the test are skill in observation and accuracy in recording. Specific guidelines follow.

Motor Behavior

    I. Activity
        A. Output—amount of activity. Is the infant very active, moderately active, inactive, etc?
        B. Tempo of movements—fast, slow, etc.
        C. Type of movements
            1. co-ordination of movements.
            2. abnormal motility patterns such as whirling, flicking, athetoid or choreiform movements, convulsive movements, etc.

    II. Mastery of Motor Skills
        A. Gross motor development — postural control, position, change, locomotion.

  B. Fine motor development – grasping and manipulation of toys, finger skills, etc.

III. Use of Motor System

  A. To approach people and inanimate objects (by position change or by reaching out).

  B. To flee from, avoid, actively ward off or get rid of a person, an inanimate object, or a painful stimulus.

  C. To express feelings—*e.g.* interest, pleasure, love, anticipation, curiosity, anger, anxiety, fear, aggression, excitement, etc.

  D. In self-stimulating activities—thumbsucking, hand play, genital play, rocking, hand-foot and foot-mouth play, head-rolling or banging, biting, etc.

Reactions to People

I. To the Parent(s)

When and how does the baby turn to the mother? What is the nature of the interchange between mother and baby? For comfort when in real distress? To share in the pleasure? Are there frequent visual, social or body contacts?

II. To the Examiner

Are there signs of discrimination of the stranger, anxiety, tentativeness in the approach? What can be said about how the baby accepts or initiates a contact; is there an attempt to engage the examiner in play? Is there behavior which could be called provocative, teasing or flirtatious? What can be seen in the facial expression, use of vocalization, motor activity, response to play and use of toys that seem to be directly related to the presence of the examiner?

Language and Communication

I. Vocalizations and Verbalizations

What sounds are heard? When? How are they used? Are there specific words? Is verbalization inhibited? Is there a change during the course of the test session? Do the sounds seem to be used in a purposive way to communicate something to another person? Are they used to express some feeling? Can the feelings be identified?

II. Non-verbal Communication

What forms of non-verbal communication are visible? How much gestural language is seen? How effective is this communication? What does the infant understand of the non-verbal communication of the adult?

III. Comprehension of Language

Does the infant indicate understanding of specific words or tones of voice of the adult? Does he associate word sounds with specific people, actions, objects or pictorial representations?

Reactions to and Use of Toys (Test Materials)

Amount of interest. Expression of preferences. How are the toys used? What is the reaction to the removal of a toy? The hidden toy? The presentation of two toys simultaneously?

In addition to the adaptive use of toys in play, does one see them being used in the service of contact with the adult? What feelings are visible around the use of toys—(pleasure, excitement, discharge of energy, aggression, anger, etc.)?

Does the baby see and hear? What is the evidence?

Changes of behavior during Test Session. Disorganization of behavior with fatigue, frustration or discomfort? Changes in mood activity or responsiveness during test?

Impressions of Parents

Interest and involvement in test. Interaction with baby. Evidences of discomfort or of pleasure. Ways of comforting infant.

Prediction of Behavioral and Personality Qualities

Although the above developmental test gives insight to the intactness of the central nervous system and the infant's psychologic status, it does not presume to predict accurately behavioral traits and predominant qualities of personality. This is so because in addition to the biologic, a host of socio-cultural and psychologic factors expected and unexpected increasingly affect the growing organism. One cannot predict either, at the time of their occurrence, whether certain events will prove specifically harmful to a child's later development. Although an early psycho-pathologic condition may foreshadow later mental illness, some of it may have beneficial influence, as when sublimation enriches the ego. Not infrequently the artist is most creative at the time of his greatest emotional upheaval. In certain children of high artistic and creative endowment therapeutic preventive action is viewed by many to carry the risk of "nipping their talents in the bud."

Thomas, Birch and Chess studied a number of children over several years and found that each infant had an *individual pattern of primary reactivity* which persisted through the first 2 years of life. They were particularly interested in an infant's reactive pattern to new situations as feeding, bathing and toileting. They found that although the primary reactive style varied in each child showing positive or negative, rhythmic or arrhythmic, mild or high intensity reaction, it remained a primary reactive characteristic of that child.

They also found that all infants do not respond in the same manner to a given environmental influence, such as child-rearing by parents. The characteristic reactions of the child and the feelings of the parents as expressed through their care, determine an infant's functioning in feeding, sleep routines, bathing, interaction with parents, siblings and in situations of special stress such as illness, or abrupt shifts in geographic environment. In this sense one can say that elements of "personality" are already present, at least in embryo, later to be more exactingly shaped by the socio-cultural-psychologic environment.

If borne in mind, this should help pediatricians to guide parents more accurately in child-rearing. If a mother understands the life style of her infant, and if it is possible for her to mesh her own personality into that of her baby's, child-rearing should proceed with a minimal amount of difficulty.

For example, the decision whether feeding can take a permissive or scheduled approach should rest on criteria beyond the pediatrician's philosophy or the mother's inclinations. Since the infant's own style of life will play a role, ideally efforts should be made to integrate realistically his pattern with that of the mother. To satisfy the needs of a baby with a rhythmic biologic time-table requires certain well defined and regularized care, rather than irregular, ill-defined and sporadic approaches. The mother whose personality is extremely casual with regard to time and schedule will obviously tend to miss or not respond to this baby's need cues. Conversely a baby with easy distractability and easy adaptability would fit more naturally to this mother's personality and there might be no problem. In brief, a crying or distressed baby may be the outcome for a mother who does not mesh with or understand her infant or his modus operandi.

Pediatricians can help a parent by explaining that even the newborn already has his own particular and primary way of reacting; his own "personality" if you will. The pediatrician can call attention to various aspects of the child's behavior which will help the parents identify his distinctive reactive pattern. What is his immediate behavior in waking, sleeping, feeding, playing; his reaction to the initial contact with people, toys and situations; his adaptability or lack of it to new food, noises, mother substitutes, changes of sleeping and eating arrangements? Important to determine also is the intensity of reaction to sensory stimuli such as those of wetness, hunger, and bowel discomfort. The quality of his prevailing mood, his attention span and persistence, and his distractibility represent other areas for making a personality inventory of an infant.

A record kept of the characteristics of primary reactivity in infants is particularly helpful when parents bring their preschool children to the pediatrician because of behavioral disturbances. Maladaptation of children is frequently expressed as defensive reactions to inappropriate parental handling. When one is able to determine the primary behavioral characteristics of a child beginning with infancy, and the manner of the child-rearing practice invoked, one may frequently trace the genesis of a problem retrospectively. The maladaptive pattern in many cases represents a caricature of the premorbid pattern. Fortunately there are other instances of incipient problems, or those just beginning, where guidance by the physician has minimized conflict and facilitated the mutual adaptation of child and mother.

The direction of behavior, so-called normal or deviant, cannot be precisely predicted inasmuch as the nature of the environmental influence plays an important part along with family attitudes and parental handling. However, the primary patterns often are persistent and this fact may be used to help parents anticipate to some extent the nature of the child's reactions and development in the preschool and early school years.

Research Possibilities: The use of prediction as one of the valuable methodologic tools in clinical child development research has come into greater prominence in recent years. In systematic, longitudinal studies of the developing child specific expectations about the course of the various aspects of development (intellectual functioning, adaptive abilities, potential problems) are measured against existing theories and practical knowledge about the current situation, status, and pre-history of the child. These expectations can be stated as predictions of various types (short term, long term, general, specific, etc.), together with the reasons for the prediction. Experiential variables considered in the context of a specific child's individual environment and his phase of development can be linked predictively to possible or probable specific effects upon development.

The outcome in children studied over a period of time makes possible the evaluation of predictions with such questions as: Did a particular prediction prove to be correct or incorrect, and why? Could a more accurate prediction have been made? What other data would be required to do so? What relevant influences could not have been predicted in this case? The advantages are evident of studying data and conditions that allow correct predictions. Examination of incorrect predictions also has demonstrated value in opening up new avenues of investigation.

Chapter 9

THERAPEUTIC MANAGEMENT

Holism is the Goal

Psychologic pediatrics encompasses comprehensive medical care of the child in the context of his family and community. It includes every aspect—somatic, intellectual, social and emotional. To be effective, the psychotherapeutic role of the pediatrician must be broad; the methods of helping must be flexible and appropriate to the varied needs of his pediatric patients. The aim is not the reconstruction of personalities, nor the impossible goal of forever irradicating symptoms. The human personality is not a slate that can be wiped clean with a swipe of the cloth. Failure to recognize this leads to unrealistic expectations and inevitable frustration.

Since psychologic pediatrics concerns itself primarily with the whole person and the whole family unit, management of psychologic problems entails involvement with the whole person and his family group, more than with a symptom or a disease as an entity. The sick "people," rather than the "disease" by itself, occupy the central position of the doctor's attention, even when the sick patient has a physical illness. The maximal auspices for such an approach would be a continuing relationship with the individual and the family group from as far back as pregnancy or the earliest years of the child. On the strength of such familiarity the doctor already has a basic knowledge and longitudinal perspective on the family and of their relationship. Where this does not exist, however, the physician must give more time and effort to enriching his store of knowledge about the child and family and their development.

The nature of all doctor-patient relationships is a two-way interpersonal reaction and communication system. It is the key to the successful management of emotional disorders. With this in mind the physician planning a regimen thinks first of realistic goals. The short-term goal for the first interviews may be only the temporary alleviation of anxiety. The longer-term goal may be the change of an attitude or technique of child care through the development of insight. Another long-term goal would be the lessening of anxiety which results from a healthier way of life.

In most instances it is wise to aim at intermediate goals—more than symptom relief, but less than total "cure." That is to say, an attempt should be made to improve the functional capacity of the patient. To the non-psychiatric physician, even less than to the psychiatrist, is given the power basically to change the personality of most people. Although all of us would hope for this power, the most we are able to do is to help a patient rearrange his life, set new goals, apply new methods, and then to live with the results.

What can the physician do? In planning management, the physician will already have assessed the nature and extent of the problem, something of its dynamics, and by his personal relationships with the parent and patient he will have used it optimally to help them psychologically. In this he will have used imagination, feeling, intuition, common sense, blended with technical skill and experience. He now faces the question of what he should do more specifically and individually to assist further the people who have come to him.

While the general rubric of "psychotherapy" covers every element of helping, there are certain elements which are particularly influential in the hands of the non-psychiatrist as well as the psychiatrist. These include teaching, educating, reassuring, clarifying, supporting, encouraging, even exhorting. It may involve changing the social and physical milieu of the patient as well. In other words psychotherapy embraces any effort to influence beneficially human thought, feeling or conduct by precept, example and personal involvement. In the broadest possible use of the term this includes "lifting of the spirit."

In pondering steps in treatment, the physician is aware of his limitation of time. For the most part, therapy must be practical and brief, although this does not necessarily mean only one or two visits. It usually involves dealing with one person primarily. The physician must decide how, when and where treatment should be given (as mentioned previously) and which one of the family group is primarily the person with whom he should deal. Having answered these questions, the physician will then proceed with what he thinks is most appropriate for him at that time.

Common Errors in Pediatric Management

1. Interviews which are delayed, hurried, or foreshortened.
2. The failure to determine who has the problem.
3. The failure to identify the primary problem.
4. The incomplete or inadequate collection of data.
5. The superficial or inaccurate interpretation of data.

6. A narrow view of etiology.
7. Communication which is faulty or non-developed.
8. Goals which are unrealistic, and treatment which is unnecessarily prolonged.
9. A loss of objectivity.
10. The failure to empathize or appreciate feelings of the patient.
11. A moralistic, authoritarian, judgmental or didactic attitude.
12. The lack of knowledge about normal developmental phases of children and adults.
13. The failure to appreciate normal and deviant mechanisms of behavior in infancy and childhood.
14. The substitution of theoretical explanations for practical assistance.
15. The failure to understand pediatric limits; the failure of referral when necessary to other resources; or the inappropriate referral.
16. The failure to prepare for referral.

Individual Help (For either parent or child)
Ventilation of Feelings

Every intelligent human being needs opportunity to release feelings. If appropriate avenues for such release are not open, they find escape in self-defeating ways. There is no substitute for the experience of being able to "talk out" feelings and attitudes. It is an area where the able physician can best serve.

Most parents come to express a variety of feelings about their children, their spouse, themselves and others. They come to complain, to criticize, to plead guilt, and in a way, to ask for forgiveness. Children also come for similar reasons; to complain and criticize parents, teachers, siblings; to express hostility and even to admit self-defeat, inadequacy and guilt. This is particularly true of older children and adolescents. Such ventilation does not always accurately pinpoint the seat of disturbance, and it may not always be candid. In fact, some feeling or attitude might be stressed which is really a mask for another more complex and unconscious one.

The physician's task is infinitely easier if the feelings are ventilated. But when there is hesitancy to express, inability to verbalize, resistance to divulge, then the physician's problem is greatly intensified and his resources are tested. If he has listened carefully in collecting the data, he may prompt the patient, but he does not prod. He can use various productive remarks such as "I imagine that it must be disturbing that Johnny still wets," or "You seem anxious that Mary isn't learning." If the patient is so bottled up that release is impossible, the physician may set another time for discussion, in the meantime doing his best to be supportive and reassuring. Knowing what to say, when and how to say it is as necessary to the medical practitioner as it is to the psychiatrist. In some respects it is more so because the physician is expected to be a "doer" in practical terms. The pediatrician can be comforted by the fact that his relationship with the child and his family is a continuing one and what has been started can develop and be elaborated in regard to the sharing of feelings, fears and anticipations.

The "doing" is not an uncomplicated task for the physician. In suggesting, advising or prescribing specific practical steps for the patient the physician must use caution. He must be reasonably sure of his recommendations and they must also be within the ability range of the patient. In his zeal to open channels of communication the physician should not substitute his own version of the problem supplying the plot of the case as he sees it. It is not the doctor's feelings and attitudes which need ventilation but the patient's. Some of the techniques of facilitating ventilation for the child have been discussed earlier (Chapter 8, Communication with child, pp. 152–153). In many respects it is less difficult than with the adult. The child has fewer societal barriers to uphold and he is less experienced in withholding. With the autistic or withdrawn child the physician may need to collaborate with his colleagues in the field of psychiatry.

Reassurance

The physician will already have provided some measure of this when he treated the patient with concern, with interest, and by competent examination. But reassurance is composed of many elements and careful thought must be given to what will reassure this particular individual in the context of his particular circumstances. What is reassuring to Mrs. Jones may be quite the opposite for Mrs. Smith. Even the use of certain words may have charged meaning for Mrs. Smith, but may be reassuring to Mrs. Jones. Hence the physician must have, by this time, some considerable understanding of the patient and the problem before he can be selectively reassuring.

Telling a patient not to worry, that "it's nothing," and urging that he give up his irrational fears and anxiety is of little value. Better than this is the technique of leading the patient to his own reassurance by virtue of the doctor's analysis of the problem and its history. It is not unusual then for the patient to come to the conclusion that "I see now that my child is perfectly normal and I have no need to worry. Maybe I need to take hold of myself." This may then lead to a consideration of how this might be done. Hopefully the doctor directs his attention to those services which can provide counselling or direct psychotherapy.

Children too can attain self-reassurance from skillful discussion by the doctor, according to their level of comprehension. The physician knows that progress has been made if a child concludes with relief that "I get a stomachache when I don't want to go to school. I think I can try going to school again." Reassurance can be a particularly useful tool with children because acceptance and approval are basic to a child's needs and serves a highly therapeutic function.

Reassurance may include an encouraging remark or an honest "pat on the back" which rings true to the patient. But if it is not done discriminately it can serve an opposite purpose. For example, telling a parent that he couldn't possibly be acting this way in view of his intelligence and personality is hardly reassuring to feelings of guilt and failure. Similarly it is not reassuring to a child to be told "You're too smart not to do well in school."

Successful reassurance creates an atmosphere of confidence in the patient, which in turn has a chain effect on the entire family organization. This requires understanding of the patient's specific anxiety and his style of behavior. Only then can the physician know what is confidence-inspiring to this particular patient in these particular circumstances, because it is based on the realities of the situation and the person. The patient is hardly convinced by the superficial, though well-intentioned, "I know you can do it."

Reassurance is nurtured by a physician's demeanor, by the way in which he explains the results of tests, by the way he helps a patient to rearrange his own life without feeling inadequate and unnecessarily guilty. The doctor must keep his evaluation within realistic limits and impart only that degree of hopefulness of which he himself is convinced, fortified by ancillary investigation. Fortunately, in most instances, the nature of the problem and the character of the parents permit him to accentuate the positive elements and to honestly encourage greater self-confidence. Suggestion is useful if it complements reassurance on realistic grounds but is not a substitute for reassurance.

Sometimes reassurance is fleeting because the anxiety is so great, or because it is "free floating," shifting from one focus to another. Suggestion is a powerful mechanism to inspire faith, hope, self-confidence and trust in a patient and is a valuable item in the repertoire of the physician. But suggestion carelessly used or when relied upon merely as a mystical force results in short-lasting relief of anxiety. Reassurance may also be transient if through the *power of suggestion* it raises false expectations, when it is not reinforced by more realistic reassurance or by some effective action.

A common error of the pediatrician is to talk too much, to reassure too frequently, to oversell the patient on what he should be like. It is a safe rule not to make statements which are not defensible. Furthermore, a good rule to follow is that of withholding information which would unnecessarily burden the patient, have no positive value for him, and serve only to relieve the physician's anxiety about possible future criticism. Too frequently, pediatricians insist on repeated examinations, though aware of the risk of so doing, for fear that their professional standing depends on having ruled out every conceivable kind of disease, however rare. In the final analysis it is worth remembering that the medical practitioner as able clinician, not as technician, makes the final decisions in handling patients, and that much in the practice of medicine depends on his skill in diagnosing even with incomplete evidence. It should be emphasized again, that basic reassurance stems from the patient's conscious and unconscious awareness of his own strengths, from the integrity, competence and sincerity of the physician, and from the working alliance established by doctor and patient.

Advice

The question of situational advising, as distinct from medical advising, is a delicate one for the physician, although the non-psychiatric physician has more latitude than a psychiatrist. The latter tends for good reason, but sometimes for what appears to be undue reticence, to give little advice or make few suggestions. The underlying factors for such reluctance have pertinence to the pediatrician as well. By advising the patient to handle a situation in a particular way, the patient may be denied opportunity to accept responsibility for his own actions or to learn to cope with them appropriately. In his dependence on the physician, no basic changes in his emotional pattern are effectuated.

Often such advice is neither good nor bad, but is simply out of place. Occasionally it is dangerous as when a physician advises a parent to have another baby in order to cement a marriage; or urges someone to marry or get a divorce for therapeutic benefit. Decisions on these matters are beyond the realm of the physician. One who takes it upon himself to act so omnipotently may do a lasting disservice to an individual. It is true that patients try to trap one into making decisions for them because they fear decision-making and feel inadequate. One danger of advising is that the physician may fail to recognize the psychopathologic condition to which he is catering. What he should do and may do with effectiveness, is to help a patient explore his situation and out of this come to his *own* decision. A doctor may be pressed to be aware of or declare his own values, attitudes and beliefs, but when he does express them, he must be sure that he does not inflict them on his patients. Even when the advice to be given is appropriate the physician may be in doubt, because it involves an attitudinal change. In such instances it is usually best not to give the advice. In emergency situations where life or health is immediately involved, the physician must directly intervene. However, these are rare.

The pediatrician must and does give advice freely as he deals with matters of physical disease. He may even with logic and effectiveness advise parents and children about certain things dealing with their behavior. It is quite appropriate, and often effective, for a pediatrician to help a parent change the environment to make it less stressful. For example, too many extracurricular activities may make some children upset; advice to curtail or identify them is certainly in order. Outlining the concrete steps a parent may take in preparing a child for hospitalization is mental hygiene at its best. What makes this advice-giving laudable is the fact that the physician is basing his guidance on facts, and on knowledge that with some degree of specificity already has proved beneficial and not harmful. The doctor has not stepped beyond his medical domain, or used an authoritarian attitude based only on meager personal experience or wishful thinking.

Support

Support of the patient is another important aspect of the doctor's helping. By support is meant the encouragement which helps a patient to proceed with a plan, a change of environment, or the modification of a personal habit. It conveys the kind of approval, praise and respect which "lifts the spirit." This of course is easily accomplished when the physician is able to agree with the patient's attitude or course of action as natural and expected for the circumstances. But when the attitude or course of action is undesirable and inappropriate, the physician must find ways of altering it *without* diminishing his supportive role. This can be done by selective questions through which the patient becomes self-aware of the pitfalls inherent in his attitude or plans. By showing his interest, concern and desire to help, the supportive interests of the physician will remain uppermost in the relationship.

Insight

In this book we have often stressed the giving of insight to a person who is puzzled and concerned about behavior. The emphasis has been on the spontaneous development of insight. We have attempted to illustrate the art of promoting insight either in parent or in child by guiding him toward a self-acquired realization of the relevant conflicts, dynamics and circumstances.

The doctor trained in authoritarian tradition is tempted involuntarily to "tell the patient." One cannot give understanding to a patient if he is not ready emotionally to hear or accept it. Sometimes a doctor believes that clinical time is saved by dogmatic explanation instead of waiting for spontaneous insight to develop. In this he risks transmitting a superficial quasi-appreciation at the expense of more durable insight on an emotional plane. Parents so indoctrinated have only a spurious understanding which may defeat subsequent attempts to promote genuine insight. Furthermore, didactic statements may evoke guilt. Even when one has tactfully tried to give a parent insight about something like faulty child-rearing, he may blurt out "So you think it's my fault; that I'm to blame." This is a common occurrence. To such a comment, we usually respond with the statement that "We do not think, nor do we say, that you are at blame; but we do believe that as parents you are somehow involved in what your child is doing. It is not your *fault*, but there seems to be a relationship between your child's behavior and what you do."

A parent is prone to think that if she has contributed to a child's problem that she warrants blame and censure. Hence even a well-intentioned explanation is frequently interpreted as such. Our task is to convey an understanding to parents of how they are involved, and yet not "at fault." This can only be achieved by fostering insight from within. It involves understanding of certain derivatives of repressed material which are below the level of consciousness at the onset of treatment, but may become accessible in a psychologically permissive atmosphere. Insight imposed from without heightens anxiety and even generates resentment which stems from guilt.

There are parents who do not comprehend or fail to be convinced that emotional factors within the family, particularly in child-parent relationships, can produce emotional disorders. An effective procedure for overcoming this block, if there seems to be no contraindications such as exposure to a communicable disease, the young age of the child or separation dangers, is to admit the child to hospital for a period of planned separation. This can be done only if the ward is appropriately staffed by nurses who by experience and personality are at ease in handling such children and dealing with their parents. If the hospital staff are themselves annoyed by such admissions, it will counteract any benefit which may be derived, and even reinforce the dynamics of the problem. (See p. 208, Pediatric Hospital Care for emotional disorders.) Where it is possible to have the child ambulant in hospital and fully occupied, including going to a hospital school, the presenting symptoms are likely to abate spontaneously and without recourse to special measures.

A typical example is the asthmatic child, or one with ulcerative colitis, whose attacks are precipitated or kept active by emotional factors in the family. Hospitalization for this kind of problem represents treatment which is indirect; as does a change of home or school environment, or a separation of the child from any noxious milieu. This does not make it less important than that which involves a person directly in psychotherapy. The latter may produce more lasting benefit and have to be used to complement milieu therapy. In our experience such children often cease to have their attacks immediately or soon after admission to a hospital. This is a kind of therapeutic test and helps a parent examine the relationships between experiences in the home and the illness of the child. From this, insight may be gained which helps parents change those agents which provoke the behavior disorder.

The therapeutic gains from separation must be consolidated by aftercare which usually involves the parents and child in a program that changes their way of life significantly—a psychologic desensitization, in effect.

Clarification

This refers to helping a patient gain an adequate perspective of his problems in order that he may better understand what is involved and try to do something about the matter. Clarification consists partly of educational and partly of psychologic support. Clarification differs somewhat from insight development; the latter involves understanding at a deeper level. Clarification is concerned almost entirely with fully conscious material, matters about which it is more or less easy to speak and where there is a minimal amount of emotional blocking.

The dominant note is understanding—understanding by the patient of himself, his environment, his spouse, his children, and the people with whom he is associated. In our efforts to clarify, we direct the person to see external realities more clearly, as well as to understand his own emotions, attitudes and behavior. This understanding ranges from thinking to concrete actions, such as considering whether a child should be placed in a certain grade or a different school. Helping a child make such a change is equally important as the change itself. The parent and the child may need help in manipulating the environment, but this should not mistakenly be a manipulation of the people themselves.

Education

Parents, and also children if they are old enough to understand, often need to know the "facts of life"; whether these be about sex, normal development, schooling, or anything else. They need to be taught and given information, or re-educated when they are influenced by misconceptions and faulty information. In some matters they need direct help, such as when to set limits, when and how to discipline a child. If Johnny is impulsively compelled to hit other children, apart from understanding its basis, the parents must know the appropriate way to deal with it so that it becomes part of helping him in the long run, as well as controlling him.

A parent may need to learn precisely how to give up over-coercion in child-rearing, just as he may need help in learning how to provide stimulation and educational direction. Giving a patient insight into the causes of behavioral disorder may help him see the temporal relationships between life experiences and behavioral symptoms. This fosters intellectual insight which by itself may not be of lasting benefit, but which may be the opening wedge to attain emotional stability.

The busy practitioner is tempted to supply "educational" reading material. Books, pamphlets, films and other media of education are more useful for stimulating discussion in groups than for individual education to influence or change attitudes and feelings. Anxiety may be intensified or precipitated by reading, as when a patient identifies with a character in a book. Such a parent, unless she has ready access to the physician or someone else with whom to talk out her newly found concern, may become quite panic-stricken if left alone with her highly charged emotions.

Group Meetings

As individuals all of us engage spontaneously in self-therapy or seek help through membership in groups. We unconsciously seek out social relationships which help allay anxiety, reduce tension, and promote emotional or material welfare. Often, however, the nature of the group is such that one cannot freely express his feelings and attitudes; criticisms from one's peers often lead to increased guilt which is not dissipated as it might be. Although the social or educational aspects of such groups are important, they may not get to the core of one's psychologic needs. Hence, homogeneous groups which are arranged to deal with attitudes, feelings and emotions around specific areas of illness or behavior problems can provide more direct opportunity for helping, as when they help a person deal constructively with his guilt.

It is the emotional experience in the group which is effective in changing attitudes. Neither pediatric nor psychiatric sponsored groups expect to bring about basic changes in character or personality, although in psychiatric groups the depth of exploration of feelings is greater, and the insight which develops tends to come from exploration of unconscious conflictual material. This is not to say that the discussion always remains on a superficial level in the non-psychiatric group meetings, or that unconscious material is never explored. It is difficult to discuss highly personal matters such as parental care or parent-child relationships on a conscious plane alone. Clearly there are always strong unconscious forces in operation when discussion is carried over into feelings. Since "below the surface" feelings may be stimulated, it becomes mandatory to realize the risks as well as the advantages inherent in their operation.

While group discussion and lectures on child-rearing cannot take the place of the one-to-one relation between a woman and her doctor, they may complement it in important ways. In the case of groups for parents of sick or abnormal children, the mother has a chance to share her troubles with others. She gains immeasurably from practical and realistic help and support of fellow members and the leader; she finds solace in discovering that she is not alone with her feeling of failure, her fears, and her guilt. This can enormously lighten her burden and renew her strength. A more positive rapport is fostered with the medical and nursing staffs.

Individual pediatricians have experimented in a limited degree with forming groups of patients to discuss some aspect of pediatrics such as a particular disease, child development, education or community relations. In pediatrics it is clear that there is merit in this approach, as there is in psychiatry. However, there are differences in the aims of the pediatrician and the psychiatrist, and hence in the techniques used.

Whether the groups are fostered by pediatricians or psychiatrists, the greatest benefit which may come is from attitudinal changes in the participants. This in turn fosters improved relationships with other persons and makes life more satisfactory. Education is a secondary goal. Each profession also believes that the psychologic benefits come maximally from verbal interchange of the participants; from parent to parent, with some gain also from the interaction of parent with group leader.

The following guidelines are presented to assist a pediatrician in planning for parent groups:

1. The organizer must first determine "the purpose of the group meeting." It might be to *teach* parents about child development and child care, to *instruct* about a specific disease and its management, or to *influence attitudes*. Groups of parents of diabetic children, for example, can learn how to administer medications, prepare palatable diabetic diets, deal with emergencies of shock. Such parents may also gain from group meetings in sharing feelings of anxiety, fears, aspirations and hopes. Whatever the group, the method or the technique, it should be tested pragmatically to determine its effectiveness and its justification.

2. The mechanics of organization must be carefully considered. In terms of membership should it include both fathers and mothers, or have representatives of only one sex? The number of persons in a group is also important. As a rule, a small group of from 10 to 12 members lends itself better to informal and more intimate discussion.

The frequency of meetings, their regularity of time and the place, should be mutually agreed upon by members with suggestions from the leader. Generally the number of meetings should not be excessive if a substantial number of parents are to be reached and if it is to remain within the bounds of economic reality. The payment of fee for group services must be clearly understood by everyone at the first meeting. There is psychologic benefit to charging a reasonable fee in order to defray the expense of leadership and overhead administrative costs. These measures help inspire a feeling of confidence from planning. They also enable the program to get results in a relatively brief time. The longer the time or greater the cost, does not guarantee greater benefits.

Types of Parent Groups

Parents have met in groups for many years for a variety of reasons. Most often they have met alone or with teachers concerning education, schools and special problems relating to children. Psychiatrists have not only fostered meetings of groups for psychotherapy, but they have experimented with group organization, techniques of therapy, and the role of leaders. Although group work is far less advanced in pediatrics and general medicine, experience of this kind is not lacking. In the next years we may see a proliferation of such groups in pediatric practice.

Groups are apt to fall into two categories. One type is planned as a lecture, or series of lectures, by an expert in the field who imparts facts and gives some practical advice. Such a teaching session is likely to be followed by a question and answer period which amplifies, clarifies, cautions. A second type is a more non-structured series, where the parents themselves initiate and carry on discussion along the lines of common interest and concern. During the sessions they are encouraged to make comments and suggestions out of their own experiences. This is based on the belief that parents need ample time to discover themselves as individuals with feelings and attitudes, rather than merely as students receiving advice and instructions.

Hospital departments of pediatrics have been especially interested in and able to use group meetings for educational and psychotherapeutic benefits. At Yale, for example, a program of training for natural childbirth included meetings with groups of parents in various combinations. These started before the birth of the baby and continued for several weeks after delivery. Generally they were held eight to ten times and were limited to a maximum registration of fifteen. The aim was to help adults learn about the physiology of pregnancy, care of the newborn, developmental landmarks of the infant and the appropriate roles of parents in child care. The purpose also was to facilitate pregnancy and delivery for the mother, and to ease the role of both parents psychologically during the pregnancy, delivery and postnatal periods.

Sometimes a member left the group for 2 or 3 weeks to have her baby, then triumphantly returned to describe her experiences and enjoy a warm welcome. Mothers of "first" babies were usually in the majority, though sometimes the mother of one or two participated in the group for a "refresher." Her wider experience was eagerly sought by the novices. Sometimes a group was set up for mothers only, with perhaps one session to which the men were invited. In others there were couples throughout.

The matters most commonly discussed in our groups seemed to follow a consistent pattern. Those in early pregnancy talked about their own discomforts and how to relieve them—nausea, fatigue, depression or moodiness. Later in pregnancy there was always much discussion of infant feeding, especially breast versus bottle. Feelings of conflict, guilt or preference were aired and the mothers learned that they could be flexible without harm to their offspring. When there were no husbands present, the mothers wanted to talk about the impact of a new baby on their men. Won't a busy domesticated mother seem much less attractive? What are the dangers of "letting yourself go?" This led to discussions of the husband's feelings and his new husband-father role.

As these women neared term, the discussion turned to the discomforts of the last days. The leader showed a diagram illustrating the strains on the ligaments from the heavy uterus, explaining the backache. There was animated discussion of the merits of natural childbirth and the conditions under which it is desirable or possible. There was also a good deal of concern about the pain of labor and about how well or badly they would behave. And as usual, the question—will my baby be normal?

When present, husbands wondered how they would acquit themselves during the delivery crisis, how they could be of most help. There was much discussion whether a husband should stay on hand during his wife's labor or even during the birth. This gave the leader an opportunity to stress the acceptance of individual feelings on this matter, as well as the hospital regulations and the doctor's preference. In summary, the expectant parents gained enjoyment in anticipation of this new experience, and greater self-assurance which comes from feeling more in control of what lies ahead. Doubts and puzzlements were clarified and the discovery made that trepidations are similarly shared by all. They learned too that there is more than one "right way" to be a mother and that they can be themselves without fear of costly mistakes.

Types of Children's Groups

Some hospitals which provide care for adolescents in special clinics have organized meetings of adolescents, similar to adult groups. However, these adolescent groups are not primarily aimed to foster change of attitudes but more to elicit expression of feelings, from which is gained greater awareness by each member as an individual, and as a member of the peer group.

Such adolescent groups too must have experienced, competent and well-trained leaders who understand adolescents, the dynamics of group interpersonal exchange and particularly the relationships of the individual to his personal environment and to society at large. The participants are concerned not only with their feelings about themselves, but about their relationships to other people, to vocations, to societal change, education and religion—in fact any area of life in which they develop stress in attempting to cope.

The role of the non-psychiatric physician may primarily be to help his adolescent patient find an appropriate group and to help him gain admission. He can also fill the role in the group, as the expert to talk about physical illness, physical development, sexual behavior, venereal disease, contraception and drugs. Not only should he be competent to talk about these subjects, but he should feel comfortable in sharing with the group leader the role of helping the participants express feelings and attitudes. Such multidiscipline and joint endeavors in group work require planning and preparation, wherein the physician meets with the group leader beforehand to learn what his exact role is to be and its limitations. Even a well-informed physician can be detrimental to a group by not understanding the psychologic implications of his teachings.

It is not customary for children of school age to meet with non-psychiatric physicians in groups for education or for expression of feelings. But psychiatrists in child guidance clinics frequently work with groups for these purposes.

More has been done in organizing groups of pre-school children. Sometimes this consists of children who are patients in hospital and come together in a nursery school atmosphere. Through play they may act out some of their impulses and feelings which have arisen out of the hospital experience. Some hospitals have set up special nursery schools for their ambulant out-patients. Increasingly day care centers or nursery schools for normal children are willing to admit one or two children to their groups in order to help with special problems. For example, children who are excessively shy or frightened may be helped by contact with such a group if the teachers are able to give the particular attention that is needed. Occasionally seriously ill children with conditions like autism are admitted to membership in a nursery school of normal children. It is even likely that such children are first detected when they have been enrolled as normal children. Often special groups of these children in a traditional nursery school, manned by teachers knowledgeable in ways of helping the deviant, are practical and of educational benefit. The parents feel "something" is being done, and the separation even though brief affords them a respite from arduous child care.

Group Leadership

Leadership of the group is an important consideration. A qualified leader may be a physician, nurse, psychologist, educator, or social worker; occasionally a specially trained lay person. But beyond training and knowledgeability in their own fields, they must genuinely like parents and be able to sympathize with their problems. As a rule, the leader should be experienced in group dynamics, as well as competent in the profession he represents. He should know how to reach the most difficult and disturbed in the group with consideration and support, how to put complex matters into simple down-to-earth terms without violating the truth—and to translate theory into practice. He must have a keen ear for "the question behind the question," for the unspoken concern which the questioner is unwilling to express or of which she is only half aware. All of this is no easy task. It takes much experience and special training in the art of leading groups. Occasionally, among intuitive professional people, there are "naturals" for the job. But many an otherwise distinguished psychologist or physician honestly recognizes his own unfitness for this work.

Leadership of the group and the leader's role should be firmly established. Sometimes a likely candidate is a parent who has gone through the experience of having a sick child, one chronically ill or mentally retarded. Even so, a professional or trained person must provide supportive leadership and bear the ultimate responsibility for the group's direction. If discussion is to focus on hospital management, nursing and medical procedures, the leader must be one who not only understands the techniques used, can describe them competently, but can also help the parent accept emotionally the regimen which is described.

The leader must be aware of the nuances of feeling within the group and must know how to deal with emotions expressed. For example, criticism may be expressed mildly or even laughingly, but it may be angry and personal. Remarks not only may be made about physicians, hospital, nurses but also may be turned on other group members as well. There may be expressions of guilt and confessions of mistakes with highly charged emotion. The leader must be able to deal with these at the time they are expressed and help direct them into fruitful channels.

Many parents, particularly at the beginning of the group meetings, have hesitancy in expressing themselves. Many of them have been non-verbal for long periods of time. The leader must know how to encourage verbal expression and to promote interchange between participant members. There are typical "openers," statements explaining the variety of feelings which parents have, ways in which children develop or react to stress, anecdotes with which the parents may easily identify.

The objective must be realized. To provide the greatest benefit for attitudinal change, the discussion technique must promote participation by the parent. To be effective, learning cannot be passive. The involvement must not be mechanical or primarily intellectual, but also personal and emotional since attitudes, prejudices and feelings are not rooted in logic but in emotions.

The parent must understand that he is free to express his hopes and fears, discuss his worries, relate his experiences to a group of peers who are interested and sympathetic because they are in the same situation. Participants must understand that the purpose is not to teach them to be good parents or necessarily to be instructed in specialized techniques. Most parents have an adequate fund of information, or know how to obtain it; what they lack is the ability to put into effective use what they already know, and how to utilize and enjoy their existing capacities for parenthood. A successful group nurtures the potentials of each person as an individual. As parents face themselves with courage, explore their own experiences, their subconscious as well as conscious needs and conflicts, they arrive at new approaches to the child because they have been liberated from blind spots and have changed attitudes which are more important than the attainment of intellectual understanding. These are the prime objectives of parent group meetings.

Family Unit Counselling

It is generally accepted that the contemporary American family is undergoing a remarkable transformation. The direction of change, regardless of class of origin, is toward the standards and expectations of the middle class. Although economically more secure, many families seem no happier for their accumulation of material things. The trend is to divest the family of many traditional work tasks; devotion to orthodox religion, care of the elderly, and responsibility for education within the home. It is believed that changes within the family basically result from industrialization, urbanization, the advance of technology. As expressions of the process of change, we frequently see family breakdown even though this is not always overt. Whether clearly evident or not, such family disorganization, often a "family neurosis," reflects itself in the behavior of children. For these problems the family inadvertently requests assistance, primarily for the child.

Since the family relationships as a whole are involved, it has become clear to physicians, whether psychiatrists or not, that there must be a diagnostic assessment of the family as an entity in the treatment of behavioral disorders in children. Frequently there is merit in dealing with parents and child (and sometimes siblings) simultaneously as a unit. Accordingly, suggestions are made that the family meet for two or three sessions with the physician, or someone he has chosen in his stead, "To talk about the family in order to get some clues to the child's behavior." The visits are usually of 40 to 50 minutes' duration, spaced at intervals of more than 1 week. Follow-up talks afford chances for a more detailed evaluation and for sustained efforts at changing attitudes and milieu. Parents can absorb and test out concepts. Accepting and rejecting suggestions, they can consolidate constructively those changes which have helped most. The series is followed in 6 months by a return visit to note progress.

The room where the family and child meet should be convenient for talking together, where the pediatrician may observe the modes of expression of parents and child in interaction with each other, and with themselves. There should be play materials and room enough for the child to get involved with them, particularly if he is too young to enter into the conversation. The parents are encouraged to talk about the child, the family, their problems, feelings regarding each other and any other topics which seem pertinent. The aim of the meetings is expressed by the physician as one of helping parents arrive at problem-solving together.

The advantages of a family unit interview is that it often provides rapid identification of "the patient" and of the problem by the family members themselves.

Most mothers welcome a chance to meet in a conference with their husbands. Despite occasional resistance of one or the other parent (often the husband) to a joint meeting with the physician, it is not uncommon that each soon becomes engaged in conversation and frequently there is an unexpected discharge of feelings about matters where there had been a conspiracy of silence. It is a surprise for each to find that their carefully guarded secrets have been known or accurately surmised by the other all along, and it is a relief to be able to discard the wariness and to discuss matters openly. Although defensiveness and hostility may be expressed at this time, these attitudes often diminish or terminate as there is a shift towards each other of sympathetic concern.

While the discussion may remain focussed for quite a time on past events and experiences which have never been forgotten, the helping goes forward if it is centered particularly on the here and now of emotional interaction between the parties. The physician conducts himself as an observant listener who by an appropriate question now and then emphasizes a point, particularly as it seems related to the parents' feelings and attitudes in child care. As parents gain knowledge of their influence on causing behavior, and are able to change their attitudes and modes of dealing with themselves and the child, there frequently is a change of symptoms.

Even when individual symptoms do persist, they may lose some of their pervasiveness of setting up hostility reactions in parents or other members of a family. The parents are able to deal with the symptoms more realistically, despite their continued involvement. The roles of the parents and child in a continuation of the emotional disorder may be more clearly recognized so that the necessity for individual therapy of one or the other is evident to the physician and to the parents as well. This facilitates referral to a child guidance clinic or to another kind of psychiatric service for specialized intensive attention.

Some pediatricians have taken special training courses in child and family behavior, and group work. The Tavistock Clinic in London has offered a variety of training programs for non-psychiatric physicians in which as participants they experience many of the interacting forces that their patients do when treated similarly in groups. What amounts to a group training experience then becomes a group learning or group therapy experience. Social workers and psychologists have similarly been trained in dealing with small and large groups for a variety of purposes. Where physicians are incapable for one reason or another of conducting family unit counselling, such auxiliary professional persons may serve instead.

Family unit counselling not only provides a medium for study of problems and conflicts of a family, but also helps the family become acutely aware of *their* resources for dealing with *their* problems. Parents often do not recognize their own strengths or the opportunities readily at hand for helping themselves. By supporting their efforts and giving understanding that family tensions are not solely of their own creation but are symptoms of modern life stress, they are helped to solve the discrepancy between some of their unreal family ideals and the actualities of modern life. From this comes greater ability to adapt as individuals to their family roles and family functions.

The Harris Family: *Effect of Non-communication Among Members*

An example of successful promotion of family unity through a single family meeting with the non-psychiatric physician is that of the Harris family. Mrs. Harris complained frequently to the physician about the rebelliousness and lack of self-control of her two sons, aged 6 and 8 years. Their behavior seemed to originate after a move from one part of the city to a more desirable and higher-rent area. Soon after this change of environment, the father began to have less contacts with his sons. He worked not only the usual 5 days a week, but began to leave home early each Saturday and Sunday morning, not returning until late at night. The boys missed the recreational periods of week-ends and even the casual contacts on school days. Mrs. Harris felt that she was left alone to rear her children and condemned her husband for his lack of understanding. After the sons had been examined and found normal and healthy, various suggestions were made to the mother about providing substitute recreation, particularly that which brought the boys in contact with men at a YMCA. But this practical suggestion proved not very helpful. The behavior of the boys continued unchanged both in the home and in school.

It was decided to invite the father, the sons and the mother for a meeting with the physician. When this was held, mother and sons soon launched into criticisms of the father, his lack of attention to them, his increased absences from the family, and his seeming disinterest in them. The father sat speechless for quite a time, but became obviously disturbed when the older son blurted out that he had followed his father one Saturday morning and found him taking a subway train elsewhere than his usual work destination, presumably to "some place where he could have fun." Mrs. Harris angrily denounced her husband as a man who had become selfish, possibly interested in another woman, of spending time with cronies at a racetrack. Mr. Harris then became agitated and heatedly answered, "All right. You have driven me to it. I will now tell you where I spend my Saturdays and Sundays. When we moved, I found that I could not meet our bills and decided I needed to have extra work. I found a week-end job but didn't tell you about it because it was work as a janitor. I did not want my wife or children to think of me as a janitor. It isn't that I didn't think or worry about you, only that I was ashamed and didn't want you to think I had failed as a husband." For several minutes there was silence, then Mrs. Harris began to weep, and both boys ran to their father, who now had also begun to sob. Soon all were crying, but there was an overtone of relief. With help, the father was able to find a different job which paid as much and gave him more free time on weekends. He used this to be with his family. Six weeks after the interview Mrs. Harris reported that "things are much better all around. We are ashamed at what happened but we are very proud of him."

Genetic Counselling

With the explosion of knowledge about heredity and inherited diseases, parents have come in greater numbers to physicians for advice about the risk of having children. Some come with questions about marriage and many seek relief from anxiety about the health of their children. The physician facing the problem of treating a child for an inherited disease also wonders how to deal psychologically with him and his parents. What should they be told about the hereditary aspects? How and when should they be given information? Social agencies not infrequently refer patients for genetic counselling or for advice in eugenics. It is evident from the large number of patients that most of the counselling could never be done by geneticists alone.

The pediatrician singly or as a member of a team with geneticists will be called upon increasingly to tell parents about genetic risks, and to provide information about the causes of particular diseases. In order to counsel competently the physician should have training and experience in the field of genetics, particularly if this includes the management of clinical problems. Such training should provide a proper understanding not only of the meaning of risk data, of probability, but also of the psychological, ethical and legal issues involved in giving genetic information.

The primary role of a genetic counsellor is to present accurate genetic information. The manner in which this is presented requires caution, tact and awareness of all the issues which are pertinent. There are many possibilities of error in interpreting genetics and giving eugenic information and advice. Even the most competent counsellors admit that genetic counselling remains imperfect. In order to help a parent, or an unmarried person coming for guidance, the counsellor should be aware of the facts and aware of their imperfections. If a specific patient is the reason for seeking counsel about his care and rearing, and the risk of having other children similarly afflicted, two factors must be considered by the physician. First he must be sure that the patient has been accurately and comprehensively evaluated genetically and medically. Second he must be aware, as far as he can determine, of the psychologic nuances which bring the questioner to him.

Genetic counselling can never involve a detached or intellectual presentation separate from existing circumstances or dealt with impersonally. The counsellor should not take for granted that people can attain a realistic attitude simply by being told the facts, however accurate they may be. This means that there is always need for a combination of giving information and personalized guidance in medical-genetic counselling. The counsellor must work through the usual doctor-patient relationship. However intelligent, the person seeking advice must be given explicit interpretation of any figures which are used. Telling a parent that the risk of having a deformed child is 1 in 4, often has been interpreted as meaning that every fourth child will be afflicted while the others in between are somehow protected. People with genetic problems, even the best educated, require instruction in the management of family problems and help to deal realistically with them. Proficiency of counselling proceeds only when there is an understanding of human psychology. Thoughtless remarks as well as scientifically inaccurate information may have a devastating effect on persons, not only in enforcing feelings of despair, but in leading them to a way of life which is unnecessary and even inappropriate.

One must be reminded that empiric risk figures are essentially pragmatic probability statements based on accumulated medical statistics. The figure employed for any specific defect encompasses a number of different etiologies. Inheritance is only one of these factors causing a pathologic condition. For that reason, these figures must always be considered tentative; revisions of such data are always being made. Admittedly a carefully taken family history highlights or delineates high risk families, even more than do empiric risk figures.

Physicians counselling a person genetically should protect themselves against distortion by keeping written records of what is said. All correspondence about patients should also be kept in copied form in order to avoid misunderstanding and even lawsuits. In dealing with social agencies, a privileged communication with the patient must be honored whether the transmission of information be written or verbal. Written consent of the parties involved must always be obtained before sending the information to a third party.

Play Activity in Pediatric Practice (Diagnostic and Therapeutic)

The physician's skill in introducing appropriate toys and play activities to relate to and communicate with many of his younger patients is a major pathway to the goal of effective assessment of these children. Furthermore, in children with psychologic difficulties, primary or secondary to a physical ailment, communication through play becomes one of the essential ways in which to establish an alliance with the child patient that provides a basis for helping him to overcome his difficulties.

Play activity may serve the child as a reassuring introduction to the physician, as a non-deceptive diversion to relieve the tension of waiting for the unknown or as relief before and after an uncomfortable procedure. In this way play serves as an indirect preparation for uncomfortable, frightening or painful examinations and procedures. The pediatrician should select a few toys that he can use easily with most age groups in a play contact. Thus, a rattle, a brightly colored ball, crayons, pencils and paper, a few simple puzzles and a picture book may serve most age groups when combined with the flash light and rubber percussion hammer in the examining kit. The toys should be simple and not too exciting.

In the infant the rattle can be used to assess hearing, vision and grasp at the same time as a playful atmosphere is created by the friendly pediatrician. In the older child the toys often serve also as a means of eliciting spontaneous movements and postures that permit assessments of neurologic functioning which the child cannot or will not perform on verbal request.

The toys and play become a major way of setting the child at his ease through providing an appropriate means for him to discharge tensions he cannot contain. In this way physical and psychologic phenomena important for diagnosis, can be elicited permitting child and doctor to talk comfortably about school, siblings, aspirations and the child's feelings and fears. Such play becomes the basis for tactfully conveying the pediatrician's sympathy and understanding to the child. In this atmosphere the child can listen to advice from the doctor and can raise questions and objections about his life situations and about those that relate to his health and care.

The theoretical basis for incorporating play activity in the pediatric examination and for utilizing it selectively in treatment should be understood by the pediatrician. According to the age of the child, the physician will select inanimate objects and provide an atmosphere that encourages the child to play. In such play activity the child is encouraged to express himself more fully and to become active in coping with his situation rather than being passive and helpless in the face of the medical environment which he is facing. Play activity can serve to prepare the child for what will happen as well as to help him play out and gradually overcome the difficulties he has encountered in his past.

For example, a 5-year-old boy was referred to the hospital to have a tonsillectomy and adenoidectomy because of an increasing deafness caused by chronically infected tonsils and adenoids. The pediatrician and otolaryngologist explained the operation and the hospitalization to the mother and child, encouraging the mother to prepare her son for this experience through further explanation and play activity. The pediatrician, using his own stethoscope and tongue depressor and having the syringe and other equipment available in toy form, demonstrated such preparation to the mother. An appointment was made about a week before the hospitalization with a hospital nurse to show the child and his mother through the ward to which he would be admitted for his surgery. The mother was able to answer the child's questions and to respond to his curiosity by providing him with opportunities to play out the hospitalization and surgery.

However, after the child returned home from his successful operation, he had recurrent nightmares and was reproachful because he said he did not know it would hurt so much. In a follow-up visit to the pediatrician's office, the little boy played out his understanding of the hospitalization and surgery, saying he was the doctor and doing to the doll patient what he felt had been done to him. He substituted an active approach for what had been experienced passively. Thus, in repetitive play the child transformed the frightening, painful effect of the hospitalization and surgery into active learning and mastery which were reassuring.

In another instance the pediatrician noted that a 10-month-old girl was somewhat unresponsive. He asked the mother how she played with her daughter. The mother was astounded and said that her baby was too young to play, whereupon the physician used a bell and rattle to arouse the child's interest as he held her, noting how she lateralized sound, had an adequate grasp for her age and became more playful with him. She chortled and smiled. The physician responded with smiles and pleasure and then placed her in the infant's bouncy chair which he had in his office. The mother reacted to this play-activity lesson with interest.

Through the use of a few toys (a ball, crayons and paper, and a flash light), a pediatrician set up a pleasant and appropriate atmosphere to talk to a 5½-year-old boy with enuresis. Using the opportunity to play and talk, the child was able to relate to the pediatrician comfortably and to discuss his bed wetting. The patient seemed strengthened in his determination to overcome this "babyish habit." The parents concurrently were able to clarify their own attitudes toward their son and then were able to turn over to the boy a more appropriate degree of responsibility for his bathing, toileting and care of his body.

In another instance, a 10-year-old child was brought to the pediatrician because of recurrent abdominal pain each morning at breakfast or soon after on school days. The child seemed shy though eager to please. The physical findings were normal. The physician introduced a bright red small rubber ball, and as they played catch doctor and patient talked of many things, including school and the abdominal pain. It became somewhat clear that this boy was worried about his parents. As he played he talked of their quarrels and his fear that they would leave each other while he was at school. The pediatrician referred the parents to a social agency for help at the same time continuing to see the child in play interviews that enabled the patient to face his anxiety about leaving home to go to school. He gradually learned to cope with this and developed the will to go to school. Ultimately he proved to himself in this way that there was no need to be upset.

Play activity serves as an informal instrument of pediatric evaluation and treatment when it provides the pediatrician with an opportunity to combine his skill in communication with the observation of children. When the physician speaks and comprehends the child's language it enables the child to identify with him as an important adult who protects and guides him in his growth and development. For the child play activity is often a comforting and a preferred means of exploring, experimenting and coping with himself and his environment.

Medications and Their Usage

Sedatives, tranquilizers and anti-depressant drugs have been found valuable *temporary adjuncts* to supportive treatment. An old but often true saying in pediatric practice is that parents need them more than their children. In our experience the drugs to which particular disorders have responded most favorably are as follows:

1. *Disorder*

Anxiety neuroses
Hyperkinetic syndromes (psychomotor acceleration)
Aggressive outbursts
Tics
Explosive outbursts of temper
Sleeping problems
School phobias
Acute fear (as of hospitalization or medical procedures).

Recommended Drug

Mild tranquilizers, such as Diphenylmethane derivatives, especially Benadryl; Atarax
Phenobarbital.

2. *Disorder*

Moderate or severe organic states, particularly distractibility, excessive motor activity, impulsivity, inability to concentrate; mild organic states that have not responded to Benadryl.

Recommended Drug

Meprobamate, such as Equanil and Miltown
Benzedrine.

3. *Disorder*

Overactive and distractible children who do not respond to tranquilizers.

Recommended Drug

Stimulants such as Dextroamphetamine (for its so-called paradoxical effect).

Principles to be Followed in Drug Usage

1. No drug should be employed without clear indications for its use, careful supervision of dosage, and precautions against toxicity.

2. Indications must clearly outweigh potentials for toxicity.

3. Reliance on a few drugs which are well known to the physician is better than the use of many, particularly when these are new,

untested sufficiently, or products about which the physician has little accurate information.

4. Drugs should not be used any longer than necessary. The dose should be manipulated periodically in order to determine if the symptoms are as well controlled on lower dosages. As a rule sudden and complete stoppage is contraindicated.

5. Dosage must be individualized for each patient. Children differ from adults in their response to drugs, as they do between themselves as individuals. Each drug used should be considered as a test of individual variation.

6. Psychopharmacologic medications should not be used in adolescence because of the tendency for that age group to experiment with drugs for the "kick" effect. There is danger of habituation.

7. Since drug treatment is only a part of the total treatment of the child, it should be started only after there has been a thorough study of the child and his problems plus attempts to deal with them in another manner. It is well known that medications have a placebo effect which sometimes is of greater benefit than the chemical reactions involved. The use of placebos has the advantage of avoiding toxic reactions and habituation.

Chapter 10

PARAMEDICAL SUPPORT IN PEDIATRIC PRACTICE

Modern Aids

Pediatricians aiming to practice comprehensive pediatrics frequently find themselves burdened with the many facets of pediatric workload: dealing with the physically sick, providing immunizations, guiding parents and caring for newborn babies. A distinct advantage for today's pediatrician is that the tools are at hand to relieve some of the burdens and permit him to practice comprehensive medicine.

To help meet the responsibilities of total patient care there are community resources (described on pages 206 to 208), or the services of other professional persons who are available for use in his own office. These include social workers, clinical psychologists, public health nurses and family educators. They may be employed on a part time basis, although large pediatric clinic groups have found it feasible to use full time help. The manner in which each of these professional persons is used depends on the needs of the physician, his ability and willingness to collaborate with others, the competence of his colleagues and the willingness of his patients to utilize these services.

Auxiliary Personnel

The Nurse

The nurse is the professional person most able to assume some of the physician's traditional role in the office. She can prepare patients for his consultation by taking some of the history, by therapeutic listening, and in answering questions. After the physician has interviewed and examined the patient and talked to the parent, the nurse may be of further assistance in talking to the parent, answering more questions, interpreting for the physician, and making suggestions which the physician and she have mutually agreed upon as being pertinent and helpful.

203

Children with chronic disease may require more attention than those who come in occasionally for the well-child check-up or for the treatment of acute illnesses. The physician may not be able to afford much counselling time with them, being forced to devote his efforts to management of their physical care and treatment. However the nurse may be psychologically helpful to such a child and to his parent by making practical suggestions for his general care as well as for recreation and schooling. These may also include problems of behavior and social readjustment. Sometimes her efforts forestall problems since anticipatory guidance is effective in the prevention of emotional problems as well as those of physical development and bodily function.

The nurse may serve as an observer of parent and child not only in the office, but also in the home. By witnessing the interaction of family members and noting the physical surroundings, she can provide the physician with information which gives new insight into the cause of some of the child's difficulties. Suggestions for changing the living arrangements, housing, sleeping and eating arrangements, or child discipline often are as effective as psychologic guidance. In the final analysis the nurse works cooperatively with the physician in an expanded preventive and therapeutic role.

The Social Worker

Social workers have been part of the medical team for many years and their vital contribution to good patient care in hospital settings and in agencies has been demonstrated. In the beginning, they dealt primarily with the problems of providing financial assistance and obtaining prosthetic appliances, or served as referral agents to other organizations in the community. As social workers became trained in casework and interviewing, with experience in child guidance clinics and in psychiatry, they gradually gave up the "Lady Bountiful attitude" and assumed an important role in psychologic assistance.

The social worker most helpful to a pediatrician in his work is one trained in personality development and child behavior, as well as in interviewing, casework, and community organization. She should have had broad experience in child welfare, family casework and child guidance.

The way the social worker functions in the pediatric office will vary, depending on a number of things. She may interview parents and children before or after the physician sees them. It is best if the pediatrician selects the patient, informs the parent of the social worker's function, and suggests an appointment. The patient is told that an evaluation is necessary in order that the physician may manage the problem more effectively. It is clear however that the pediatrician will carry the final responsibility for management. If a patient refuses such assistance, it should not be forced. It should be available later when the parent is more motivated to accept it.

The caseworker usually spends one introductory session with a parent, usually the mother. She may contact other social agencies or other groups who have known the patient in order to collect information. She then prepares a written report for the physician's medical record. A conference with the pediatrician indicates if the social worker should have further meetings with a parent and child. Where he feels that parent or a child needs special psychologic help from the worker, the parent is informed, and told of what the interviews will consist.

The function of the social worker with a parent depends on her training, what the pediatrician expects her to do, and what she sees as her proper role. It may be that of an interviewer; it may be to prepare the parents intellectually and emotionally to work through their own problems in a manner which fosters the development of satisfying and constructive parent-child relationships. In some cases, it may be to interpret the need for other services, particularly psychiatric. Some problems are clarified by the social worker whose skill is to evaluate strengths and weaknesses in the family relationship after they have been uncovered. In interviewing or in casework the social worker aims at a relationship which can be emotionally beneficial as well as pragmatically useful.

One or two sessions of casework interviewing with a social worker may give a patient insight into faulty child rearing, as when a parent is overstrict, coercive, or negligent. The pediatrician and the social worker may decide to recommend further interviews with the pediatrician alone. This may be to interpret medical symptoms or provide reassurance. Other recommendations may be for referral to a laboratory for examinations as an electroencephalography or psychometric testing. Some parents will accept casework therapy but not psychiatric referral.

Many patients do not care to go to a social agency for fear of intrusion on their privacy and damage to social standing. With the active support of a physician, a social worker is frequently able to help a patient because her services are an extension of an already existing service. The patient takes comfort from the knowledge that the worker is engaged in the handling of his problems in team with the physician. The services of a social worker seem logical to a parent who comes to a physician in what appears to be not only a medical crisis, but also an emotional one.

Occasionally a social worker is trained to do play therapy with children. This resembles that done in a child guidance clinic. It has merit when the social worker has had appropriate training and such clinic services are not available or are refused by a parent.

The Clinical Psychologist

Pediatricians frequently refer patients to qualified clinical psychologists for psychometric testing or for play therapy. Groups of pediatricians may find it practical to employ clinical psychologists part time to work with them in their offices. Parents frequently prefer referral to psychologists within the office rather than in a mental health center because it appears more "naturally medical". Such an arrangement also facilitates communication between pediatrician and psychologist, and exchange of information is expedited.

The psychologist from interviews and testing can determine the type and degree of a behavior problem and determine if more intensive evaluation or treatment is needed. He may discover behavior problems which a parent had not discussed with the pediatrician. The pediatrician may expect the clinical psychologist to help parents understand developmental problems, situational conflicts, and to receive short-term counselling for their problems. Psychologic evaluation by projective and intelligence tests does not take second place to such counselling, but continues to be one of the most effective contributions psychologists can make. One advantage of testing a child in a physician's office is the sense of familiarity which a child has from his previous visits. On the other hand, the child who is frightened when he comes to a physician's office will never be in a good frame of mind for testing there. The office of the physician will then be inappropriate.

The psychologist who is most helpful will be one who understands not only his own skills, but also his limitations. He is aware, as is a pediatrician, of the limitations of short-term counselling and the dangers in uncovering painful material when there are no resources available to help a patient cope with it. He must be one who has been thoroughly trained in child development, experienced in discussing problems with parents, capable of integrating the information which he has obtained and in cooperating with the pediatrician in planning for the patients. His familiarity with community resources is also essential.

Community Resources

The growing social and medical problems of today have forced an increase in community facilities to cope with them. While the needs still outweigh the facilities there are nevertheless a variety of community resources which may be tapped by the physician to augment and facilitate comprehensive patient care. Whether or not the physician has a social worker to help refer patients to community agencies, he himself should know the names, addresses, intake requirements and something about the characteristics of their services.

Agencies

Before referral to any community agency, it is well to know whether admission is likely in the immediate future. Nothing is more frustrating to a client, than being told that there is no place for him when he is highly motivated and brings himself for help. Long waiting lists discourage clients, frustrate physicians, and add to the difficulties of persons working in such organizations. The physician who refers an emotionally disturbed child must prepare the agency staff by discussing the nature of the problem, the reason for seeking admission, and the goals. The staff frequently needs explicit guidance on their expected role in augmenting pediatric care. Problems created by waiting lists can be minimized by preparing parents for the delay by offering support and guidance in the interim.

Child guidance psychiatric clinics today are increasingly family guidance organizations. Because of the great demand on their services they frequently have special requirements for admission.

Family service organizations no longer deal only with social welfare assistance, legal aid, homemaker or other "services." They are prepared also to deal with parents in psychological distress, especially where there is disunity and impending family breakdown; their intervention may help the marital situation and prevent psychosocial injury to the child.

Nursery Schools and Day Care Centers

Every physician has at least one favorite private *nursery school* that he recommends to his patients, and where he may personally serve as pediatrician. He should also be aware of the existence of other nursery schools, and particularly the *day care centers* with their specialized functions.

Schools

Parents may come to a physician for guidance about *schools*. Often they benefit most from referral to an educator in the community who is competent to advise about the advantages and disadvantages of a school placement because he is informed about the policies, staffing and programs of individual schools.

Special training schools for the care of neurologically impaired children and for those mentally retarded are often better known to physicians than are schools for healthy children. On the other hand, advances in the field of education for the handicapped are now so great that it behooves physicians to keep abreast of changes even in those resources which are considered primarily medical.

Residential Treatment Centers

Certain children need a structured setting for 24-hour care outside their homes. This is particularly true of impulse-ridden children who have been involved in dangerous antisocial acts such as firesetting, stealing, assaultive and destructive behavior. Many of these children also have severe school learning difficulties and will have been expelled from school. Often they lack an affectionate and sustained relationship with any adult, or with their peers. It is not unusual that there is a history of many foster home placements because they come from severely disorganized families.

The therapy from residential treatment comes from the total living milieu, although individual and group treatment is selectively afforded to some children. There is also assistance to their families. The group living experience provides them with the support and rules they need, as well as with a motivation for achievement. Pediatricians frequently are part-time members of the staff, while full-time workers comprise social workers, teachers, child care workers, psychologists and workers in arts and crafts. Child psychiatrists may be part- or full-time members.

Pediatric Hospital Care

For certain children who are emotionally ill the pediatric ward can offer care and opportunities for psychologic enhancement. Failure to thrive, child abuse, psychosomatic illnesses and attempted or contemplated suicide, are the conditions which have particularly benefited from collaborative pediatric and psychiatric treatment in a pediatric ward. Their parents usually are more willing to accept psychiatric help in that setting than in a psychiatric hospital.

Although such care is the responsibility primarily of the pediatric staff, collaboration with child psychiatrists, social workers, teachers and other personnel is essential. Sometimes there needs to be a modification of the ward environment in order to protect the child and help him optimally.

Admission to an in-patient pediatric service may present certain obstacles, however. Often pediatric house officers and nurses dislike the idea of admitting emotionally disturbed children, for whatever purpose, to a pediatric service. They are particularly concerned about one who is suicidal. They may contend that the adaptation of a pediatric ward for a special child will deplete the resources of ward personnel and diminish the quality of care to the rest of the patients. Parents of other patients may share in this concern. This need not always follow where staffs are resourceful.

Chapter 11

SPECIAL PROBLEMS

Autism

Strictly speaking autism is a form of thinking in which the content is largely endogenous. All persons to some degree normally engage in this kind of subjective thought. Current concepts define autism as a state where thinking and behavior are essentially characterized by withdrawal. Clinically the pathologically autistic child may be considered under two diagnostic categories, each viewed separately according to age of the patient, yet it is likely that each is related to the other; (1) infantile autism and (2) childhood schizophrenia.

Infantile Autism

Infantile autism, or atypical behavior, as the name suggests refers to *infants* with particular characteristics of introversion. Many of these babies continue to show symptoms later in life as childhood schizophrenia; some of the latter, however, may never have shown symptoms before childhood or adolescence.

The pediatrician should suspect the disorder when mothers complain of the following traits: A baby who does not relate well, who is very good but inattentive and not demanding; not interested in people, averts his gaze when facing another person at close range or seems to watch "out of the corner of the eyes", is unhappy and cries constantly, is slow in development, especially in speech, is apprehensive and has tendency to become frightened with little provocation. Many of these traits have appeared by 4 or 5 months of age.

In others, the first signs appear in the second year after a history of normal development in walking and talking, in relating to people and in demonstration of pleasure in play. The onset may appear suddenly. Words learned are no longer used; vocabulary does not increase, there is a disinterest in people, a preoccupation with self-activities and increasing timidity. They may show peculiar posturing of arms and legs, often accompanied by head-banging and body-rocking. Interest in play is limited to activities which repetitively involve moving parts of the body or in spinning objects, and in experiencing pleasure at being spinned. The placid child may now become hyperactive and impulsive. Apprehension, fear and timidity are prominent despite a paradoxical tendency to be reckless and to court danger.

The pre-school child may be mute, withdrawn, unresponsive and excessively restless. Behavior may be reminiscent of children who are mentally deficient, but again paradoxically these youngsters seem to have amazing memories plus ability to perform difficult tasks with skill and determination. They may have particular interest in music and rhythm. Those children who continue to speak use words sparingly and often do not refer to themselves as "me" or "I." Children who have been mute for several years show that they have been learning despite their silence. When they begin to use speech again, they often have an astounding vocabulary and show an amazing precision in recollecting complex activities experienced in their mute early years.

What characterizes these children is a mental condition that interferes with their normal learning in early life, and seriously blocks their emotional development. Extreme aloneness and an obsessive insistence on rituals in eating, sleeping and playing are often remarked upon by parents, as well as their peculiar posturing which may have already been apparent as babies. They appear stiff and unresponsive. They do not cuddle as most mothers wish of their babies, and they seem happiest when left alone with their own surroundings.

Although they are keenly aware of persons and objects, they seemingly disregard, ignore, and even try to exclude everything outside themselves. Paradoxically, they are frequently oversensitive to ordinary sounds. Noise upsets them, makes them restless, tearful and anxious. They press their fingers to their ears to shut out even minor sounds. They notice with apprehension the slightest change in their surroundings. Through their sensory systems, they take in a great deal of what goes on about them, yet they do not express the usual emotions of infancy and childhood.

Autistic children feel little need to communicate. Language is not a means of conversing with other people; rather it is a kind of shorthand of peculiarly metaphorical expressions which satisfy the speaker yet have no meaning, or an obscure one, for the listener. A single word, like the noun *dinner,* may be used to express many meanings. The word may represent *mother* who feeds the child, *food,* the *dining room,* the *father* who plays with the child at mealtime or something else. The pre-school child may repeat sentences parrot-like, echoing word combinations they have heard and stored for playback. They can recite rhymes, prayers, but they do this mechanically, without emotion or apparent understanding.

Their need for sameness is manifested also in rituals. Blocks or toys must be placed in the same arrangement time and time again. Should one be misplaced or out of line, the child is tearful, angry and agitated until the proper order is restored. Their memory often is phenomenal; for instance after a lapse of many days, a child may insist on the exact restoration of an arrangement of toys, even though it had no special design to the parent. Feeding difficulties are common. A new food or the use of a new utensil like a knife or fork may be upsetting.

An autistic child often relates skillfully to objects, plays happily alone with them for hours at a time, smiles at them and gets angry with them. As mentioned before, a special peculiarity is the pleasure he derives from twirling and spinning objects and from spinning or rocking himself. Rhythmic body movements put him in ecstacy. He responds with giggling and he can continue spinning indefinitely. He is indifferent to all people, parents as well as strangers, although he is aware of their presence. Certain of these children are discribed as "symbiotic" because they cling to the mother in a poorly differentiated but insistent manner. The "symbiotic" atypical child is thought to be more responsive to emotional and social stimuli and demands.

Psychiatrists differ in their ideas about the etiology of autism. Some think it is the result of infant care and child-rearing by parents who are themselves neurotic or even psychotic. While it is true that some mothers of autistic children are themselves cold, impersonal, even depressed, and find little pleasure in communicating with the children or in stimulating them in other ways, most mothers seem no different from normal women. It has been said by some observers that fathers of autistic children tend to be unemotional, perfectionistic, highly intelligent, "scientifically objective" in all their relationships with people. The best studies of personalities of parents of autistic children are those made in England by the Maudsley Hospital group; there seems to be some statistical significance that the fathers more than mothers tended to neuroticism and introversion.

Adherents to the theory that parents play a significant psychologic role in the causation of autism find support in studies of children reared in institutions and foster homes. Deprived of psychologic stimulation they showed underdeveloped and deficient egos, and in behavior resembled autistic children.

In contrast to those favoring the psychogenic origin, are those who believe that there is a biologic deficiency, some brain damage or other defect of the central nervous system, which is basically responsible. Although most of these children show little or no history suggestive of birth trauma, or of paranatal or other disease, there is resemblance between the behavior of the autistic child and those who are brain damaged. Many of the atypical or psychotic children develop epilepsy.

③   Where the opposing schools of thought come together in some agreement is in their acceptance that basically there is difficulty in the communicating systems in the patient, and between him and other people. Whether there was understimulation, inappropriate stimulation, inability to receive or perceive stimuli in the usual fashion in the critical periods of infancy, or whether the defect is in the integrative and executive functions of the nervous system, is not always readily proved. But the end result seems to produce abnormalities of *function* of the central nervous system, and an inadequate development of the ego and the concept of the *self.* Methods of treatment might be expected to be different as long as there are differences of opinion about etiology, yet there are basic similarities in therapy.

①   Those favoring psychogenesis feel it is important that the child be more stimulated by the mother or competent substitutes. They suggest that this be done by speaking to the child frequently while caring for him, by socializing with him in play, by initiating play which provides tactile and kinesthetic stimulation and promotes motor activity. Stimulating proprioception will enhance perception. Helping a child use his hands, walk and to talk, stimulates equilibrium and vestibulo-ocular responses. For the pre-school child, helping him with some concept of form, space and time gives him understanding of his environment and helps him establish a clear concept of his own body and how to master it. As a rule these children do not do well in a play space which is too great, where there are few limitations and where the child feels too unconfined. He does best, certainly in the beginning, in a structured environment, in having opportunities to relate to one person rather than to more.

②   The organicists are in agreement that these children need help in improving their perceptual motor, speech and cognitive functions in order to enhance neurologic integration at the brain stem, diencephalic and cortical levels. They suggest many techniques for helping establish space-time unity, and stimulation as well as inhibition of various nervous system centers. Some psychologists favoring the organic theory of the etiology, apply methods of therapy called operant conditioning and reinforcement. This is a means of behavior modification by rewarding a response (behavioral act) so that the probability of the same recurring response is increased. For example, giving praise to a child when he has obeyed a simple request pleases him so that he associates success with gratification and is inclined to repeat the act on other occasions. Food may be another reward, a positive reinforcer. There are also negative reinforcers which should be viewed skeptically. For example when an electric shock produces pain which increases the chance of a response recurring by its removal. Advocates of operant conditioning believe that such techniques make it possible to teach complex behavior when the modifier rewards the response which approximates the desired behavior.

The pediatrician is already aware of the use and limitations of rewarding behavior which is approved and "good." It is a technique he has advocated for a long time. The difference is that the professional person or the parent who uses operant conditioning methods applies them in a *systematic* way, *in steps*, whereby a complex act is broken down into simpler components which the child can master first and then move on. In fact, most parents inadvertently reinforce their children's behavior and help them learn by rewarding with praise and encouragement each successful step in their achievements.

For the pediatrician, the important task is to detect early in infancy those babies who seem potential risks, or already are autistic. The family history, particularly the description of the type of infant care, and the personalities of the parents may give the physician some clue as to why the baby is not developing appropriately. Even more important are those clues stemming from the mother's description of the baby's behavior.

Diagnostic study requires developmental examination of the baby in addition to the usual thorough physical examination. Appropriate measures to be taken therapeutically should include work not only with the baby, but with the parents as well. Psychiatric consultation may be helpful in planning therapy. Probably the best therapist of the baby is the mother, or a competent substitute, who can structure child-care programs appropriate for stimulating the atypical infant. Child care which is scheduled routinely but not monotonously, provided in a stable place and administered by the same devoted person, seems to make these infants more comfortable, less apprehensive, more trusting. As time goes on variations in care may be introduced advantageously.

Helping parents overcome uncertainty of what to do for and to the child is an appropriate role for the non-psychiatric physician. As he helps parents to be decisive, as he gives them clear-cut guides about discipline, helps them arrange daily activities by schedule and helps them promote consistency and constancy in child care, he reinforces positively the natural inclination of most mothers to give of themselves in infant care. Such guidance also assists parents to cope with their frightened resentful feelings of inadequacy.

Nursery school teachers and psychologists knowledgeable about these children, and particularly about play, may teach parents methods of play which are appropriate to stimulate not only for pleasure but for the promotion of learning. An environment providing heterogeneous sensory experiences promotes learning in all children, and theoretically should particularly benefit the autistic child. Also, continuing social contact along with sensory stimulation encourages learning even more.

Cognition fails to develop when there is reduced stimulation and when there is insufficient social contact.

Progress is not rapid in children who already show autistic behavior in infancy and it is more difficult to change the older child. But any strategies which help a child perceive, recognize and manipulate his environment adds to his learning, gives self-confidence and does away with anxiety since he now is more sure of his ability to predict and control the environment. The autistic child for one reason or another has withdrawn from the environment and needs to be helped to make contact with it, to realize his place in it, and to feel that he has some large measure in its control.

In summarizing, *the role of the mother* should be to assist ego and improve neurologic response. These may be accomplished by the following which apply equally to normal children:

(1) Establishing a structured child-care program in which there is a setting of the boundaries of space, time, personal role, self-care.

(2) Dealing with the child decisively, without uncertainty or apprehension as if he were fragile; this promotes self-trust and self-confidence.

(3) As far as possible dealing with the child consistently and with constancy. This reinforces his growing self-confidence and trust in his environment.

(4) Playing with the child in friendly and encouraging ways which help him feel a relationship with another person, especially in games and play which stimulate various sensory modalities and are pleasurable and rewarding.

(5) Arranging play and other experiences so they are in a space which is not boundless, yet not too constricted. Knowledge of spatial limits gives feeling of safety and protection.

(6) Talking to the child frequently, but not overwhelmingly and without coercing him to respond; encouraging his attempts at speech through responding to it as in a dialogue. Encouraging verbalization by describing the child, his body parts and the characteristics of his toys (color, size, etc.).

(7) Having rules and trying to enforce them consistently but not punitively. Such monitors from outside help a child delineate his "self." As a child realizes a separation from himself and others, he has incentive to view himslf as *separate* and as an *individual* who *"is and does."*

(8) Rewarding a child's successes with a smile or words of approval, through physical contact as with a pat on the back, or by giving him a favorite toy to play with or food to eat, reinforces his desire to achieve still more.

The prognosis of autism is hazardous. Making a prognosis of autism is dangerous since much of the outcome depends on many things; the severity of the condition, the time of its diagnosis, the treatment used.

though he retains some of his peculiar traits, and by his ability to function effectively and with satisfaction despite his lack of pleasure or social ease when he is with people.

Case of M.S., age 7 years. Autism: First recognized at school age

He was the youngest son of two children. The parents were both writers who had to struggle hard to maintain themselves and to get established. The mother had been depressed much of the time since the unplanned birth of M.S. Care of baby was mostly by sitters, and he was left to himself much of the time. Patient was referred to pediatrician by school because he seemed defective; speech was infantile; he was incontinent of urine; he had uncontrollable rage when anxious, which seemed each time he was pressed to do some school work. On beginning school he had shown an interest in play, but was much alone. He was removed from kindergarten, and rapidly deteriorated emotionally and intellectually. Speech was given up and he no longer played to amuse himself. He seemed not to notice or recognize parents or brother.

Physical examination showed no neurologic abnormalities and no disease. He was admitted to a State Training School for defective children because that was the only resource available. The psychiatric staff attributed the disintegration of ego and the reversion to primitive behavior to a failure to achieve gratification (pleasure of the self) or a sense of identity in infancy and early childhood, possibly traumatic experiences, and probably a biologic predisposition. Unfortunately, he has remained a patient in the institution for the past several years without improvement.

Suicide

Suicide is rare in childhood, although there are suicidal attempts in children as young as 8 and 9 years of age with the first peak at 10 years, but becomes increasingly common during adolescence. Suicide reaches its second peak incidence between 15 and 19 years of age when it is the third most common cause of death. More girls attempt suicide than boys.

The tendency of parents is to conceal the suicidal attempts. It is hard for them to believe that children become depressed. Often they minimize the seriousness of an attempt, or frequently deny the possibility entirely, even when children repeatedly threaten to destroy themselves. The thought is too dreaded to be entertained for long. While it is true that today the word "depression" is used loosely by many people (particularly adolescents), there is evidence to suggest that many children in the preadolescent and adolescent periods are depressed even to the point of seriously considering whether life is worth living or not. That being so, repeated expression of feelings of loneliness, unhappiness and a wish to die must always be taken seriously by parents, teachers and physicians.

Most children give such warnings, and frequently go farther (as if they were seeking help in preventing the act), when they leave notes of farewell, pay up all their debts, or announce as one boy did recently when parting from his friends, "Good-bye, I won't be around for a while." Usually such tell-tale evidence is only remembered after a suicidal attempt, when those concerned attempt to reconstruct the life experiences of the child before the event.

When a pediatrician is told by a parent or a teacher that a particular child is depressed and appears desirous of dying, efforts should be made immediately to prevent an attempt at self-destruction. Emergency psychiatric assistance should be sought. Hospitalization may be required, preferably in a place where careful watch may be provided constantly for at least several days. Observation should not be so overt and jailer-like as to upset the patient and make it appear that he was not to be trusted at all. Keeping a child busy, and having him involved with other persons, provides a more natural method of observation and of information collecting.

A tendency for parents, medical and nursing staffs is to "work on" the child for information about his motives, plans and the meaning of the precipitating factors. Tenacious interviewing, particularly by a number of persons, adds to a child's feeling of guilt and worry. They may make him so resentful and antagonistic that he is tempted to fight back in ways which would adversely effect those at whom his suicidal attempt was aimed. It is best to limit interviewing about the intimate and personal details to one person who is skilled in dealing with such patients, not only in getting accurate information, but in obtaining it in ways which are therapeutic. As a rule this will be the psychiatrist or social worker. Ordinarily such persons should not be the ones who deal with his body in nursing or medical care which may be painful or emotionally stimulating.

Wherever possible children considered suicidal, and those who have actually attempted to take their lives, should be placed on a hospital pavilion where they may be treated as children in trouble. While children may be treated humanely and with special concern on a ward which is primarily arranged for adults, there is usually greater benefit if placement is with other children, and where there is a staff which has had particular training and experience in dealing with children.

The first efforts at helping a patient who has attempted suicide should be to save his life. This may require skillful emptying of poisons from the stomach, use of respirators, the administration of fluids, and surgical intervention and repair. Children found to be unconscious or in a state of extreme lethargy, frequently present problems of diagnosis. There may be a history of head trauma, or of chronic disease, such as diabetes, in addition to the self-inflicted injury; in fact, the latter may have been a reaction to the former, but is temporarily masked by it so that emergency care is limited to treating it alone. Suspicion of a suicidal attempt by overdose of drugs should be entertained in every instance of unconsciousness or extreme lethargy when there is little else to explain it.

Administration of drugs to a disoriented child must be done with caution if at all, lest they be given to children who already are toxic from their use. Where there are delusions and hallucinations, not only should the child be protected from himself and from every kind of injury, but the content of his delusions should be noted since they may provide clues as to the type of person the child is, and the kind of experience he had which led to his disturbed emotional state.

In recovery from a suicidal attempt children react with feelings of despair, guilt, shame and resentment. Often they are frightened and confused, whether they have taken drugs or not. They seem to fear that something beyond their self-control is occurring. They may become very restless. When restraint is needed, physical restraint which does not imply punishment is more acceptable; it gives the child the secure feeling of being controlled.

The presence of a parent or other persons recognized as friendly and accepting by the patient also supplies reassurance and feelings of protection. If a parent can be in control of his emotions, and not feel the need to reproach or to ask questions of the child at that time, he is the ideal person to remain with the patient until he is better self-controlled, reassured and no longer confused about his whereabouts. As a child who was unconscious or disoriented becomes lucid, he should be told where he is, and what has happened, but probing for details concerning the event and study of the previous life history should be postponed until the child is rested, completely oriented, in contact with his surroundings, and able to participate in reconstructing what has happened.

The etiology and psychopathology of suicide usually relate to repeated stressful situations with which the child finally finds it impossible to cope. Defenses which he has used successfully up to that time seem to give way. A new or a larger burden suddenly becomes the precipitating agent. Usually these children are not psychotic, although schizophrenic and depressive psychoses leading to suicide may appear in children who are pre-adolescent and adolescent. Mentally defective children, as well as bright children, may be tempted to suicide. Imagined or real failure in school, in sports or in some other life situations, fear of parental acts and punishment, as well as misconceptions about what is happening to one's body and mind, are some of many situations with which children find it particularly difficult to cope. They try to deal with the stress in a variety of ways and this may be successful for a time. But if the stress continues or increases, their tolerance seems to diminish so that even a minor episode which is customarily tolerated, proves to be too much and makes the child feel helpless.

Death of a parent, separation and divorce always produce grief in children. Occasionally they attempt suicide not only to escape from painful experiences, but to protest or show hostility and anger. Acting-out aggressive behavior may take the form of suicide. There may be an impulsiveness in the act, with the aim to bring attention to the self, and to one's plight. Unfortunately, some children feel the need to go to the extreme of suicide in order to try to win back interest and affection of a parent or other loved one, or to unite parents who have separated.

Physicians should be alert to the possibility that a child's suicidal ruminations may be stimulated by death, especially suicide of a relative or loved friend. Anniversaries marking the death of a parent, whether by suicide or not, should be noted because they are periods when any person closely related may again experience feelings of grief, and have fleeting or protracted wishes of joining the dead person.

Opportunity for the non-psychiatric physician and the psychiatrist to complement each other's services is provided in the management of patients who have attempted suicide. The general practitioner and pediatrician are usually the first physicians to be called. It is their duty to provide emergency treatment, or see that the child is placed in the hands of a hospital staff for such care.

Referral to a psychiatrist for further diagnostic assessment regarding the psychologic background, etiology and psychopathologic condition is initiated by the pediatrician who helps the family obtain the best services available. During the period of psychiatric evaluation and therapy, the pediatrician can do much to encourage the parents, reassure them about the psychiatric evaluation and even re-interpret material which the psychiatrist tries to share with them. Parental guilt may lead to denial of their roles in causing the child's difficulty or precipitating it. Often the parents seem to be ambivalent in the belief that there are psychologic underpinnings or that the patient is in need of psychologic treatment. As a consequence, the parents feel increasingly uncomfortable with the psychiatrist. They are ashamed that he has had to be brought in and they may express open hostility to him.

If the relationship between the psychiatrist and patient develops fruitfully and the child benefits from it, parents sometimes become envious and their ambivalence may lead to termination of psychiatric help. Such termination could be upsetting, even detrimental to the child, since it removes an important and especially meaningful support. A pediatrician may be of great service to all parties concerned if he is able to protect the psychiatrist's assistance to the child.

It is not unusual for parents to worry about the possibility of a second attempt. This may lead to oversolicitous and overprotective care, attitudes which an adolescent may particularly resent despite the fact that basically he enjoys the added attention of the new relationship. Where a pediatrician continues to have close contact with the child as he provides general health care, parents often feel less alone in watching for signs of another impending crisis. This is not to say that children and adolescents, however well observed and seemingly in psychologic balance, may not act impetuously, or without much warning do things which are detrimental to their life and health. But as a rule, the pediatrician who has a close, long time, friendly and confidential relationship with a child or adolescent should be able to pick up clues about the child's reaction to stress and to those crises which seem particularly upsetting, even before the development of extreme defensive measures culminating in psychosomatic illness, neurotic or acting-out behavior, or suicide.

Where a child has been hospitalized for a suicide attempt, it may be easier on both parents and child if his return home is gradual, as when he is permitted to attend school outside the hospital during the day, but return to it at night. Long weekends at home may also be a good reintroduction to normal life and a way of desensitizing the parents to anxiety about the child's mental health.

Where disturbed family relationships continue to exist, a pediatrician along with a psychiatrist, social worker or family-care agency, may be needed for working with the parents to help them deal with their own life crises, particularly as these may involve attitudes and relationships which disturb their children.

In those cases where there has been a second suicidal attempt, it frequently is due to a failure to help the family with their problems. Sometimes this results from non-involvement of parents and child with the professional persons so that intensive work was not possible, and the basic psychopathologic condition remained unchanged. Where stress between child and family cannot be alleviated, placement away from home must be considered. Where assignment in school has been particularly stressful because it has been inappropriate for the child, a change of school or of classroom may be an important step in stopping the development of a situation which is intolerable.

The Case of B.L., age 14 years. Suicidal Attempt

   Presenting Complaint. B.L. was admitted to the hospital after he had left notes for friends saying that he was preparing to kill himself. A cache of sleeping pills was found in his bedroom. A "model child," who exceeded athletically when competing with his peers, yet who never was satisfied with his performance, particularly after he played tennis against his father. One day he injured his knee in a fall on the tennis courts. He was required to remain inactive for a few days and then a cast was applied for several weeks. During this time the boy was happier, more at peace in relationship to his father, and less competitive in his school work.

When the cast was removed and he was told that he could use his legs, he seemed depressed. He talked about changes that he thought had taken place in his knees that would require recasting and immobilization again. He predicted that he would become an invalid. His affect seemed inappropriate to the parents, who said that he seemed to enjoy the thought of being physically handicapped. When given a prognosis of good health instead, and when urged to return to school and rejoin his group in gymnasium and tennis, he developed a number of other complaints, especially pain in different parts of his body.

Discussion. Physical examinations each time revealed a child who was physically healthy but discouraged and worried. His sleep was disturbed and in his dreaming he talked aloud about the tennis coach who was "trying to kill" him. In discussing the dream the boy recalled that the coach looked like his father and that the "killing" was more defeat in playing tennis than actual murder. Restlessness in sleep and sleepwalking was soon accompanied by loss of appetite, a failure to achieve in school, and talk about the hopelessness of life. It seemed that restoration of physical health had resulted in emotional breakdown, by uncovering his preoccupation with the worthlessness of life.

It was in this setting that the parents became alarmed and informed the pediatrician, who admitted him to hospital for protection against suicide and for assessment of his orthopedic and psychologic condition. A psychiatrist saw him in the hospital frequently in order to study the severity of his depression and the depth of his suicidal impulse. The psychiatrist advised the nursing and medical staff how to manage the patient in a general pediatric ward without either adding to the anxiety of the patient or in causing concern among fellow patients or their parents. The patient continued psychiatric therapy on an out-patient basis following discharge from the hospital.

Rape

Rape and charges of rape are not numerous among children but the physician to whom such a child is brought often faces difficult decisions medically, legally, ethically and psychologically. He will want to keep the necessary examination to the minimum to avoid traumatizing the child even further. Yet, when it is probable that there has actually been sexual intercourse, the physician has the following obligations: proper collection and recording of necessary evidence and its release to the appropriate law enforcement and court authorities; reassurance and guidance for the parents since the way they accept the problem will have a definite effect on the child's long term psychosexual development; determination of possible pregnancy, venereal disease, or other infection calling for treatment.

The routine usually used is: (1) consent is obtained for physical examination, the collection of specimens, and the release of information to the proper authorities. (2) A careful history is taken in the exact words of the individual, giving full particulars as to time, place, alleged assailant, and other pertinent information. (3) In the physical examination of the victim, special attention is given to traumatic lesions of the body or genitalia. Disturbances of clothing, hair, etc., are noted and specimens are collected. (4) Laboratory studies include examination of vaginal aspirate for sperm in a wet preparation and also examination in a stained smear. Smears and cultures for gonorrhea and serology for syphilis are done as indicated. In the case of a girl past puberty, he must determine whether there is a pregnancy and if so, how he should proceed according to his conscience. Since the law or religious teachings or both may be in conflict with his conscience, this is not an easy decision.

When a child is violently upset following the attack, a coherent account of what has occurred can hardly be expected. She needs immediate reassurance and the presence of sympathetic and familiar people, first and foremost her parents. Rest, usually calling for sedation, is in order. While on-the-spot questioning, before a victim has had a chance at second thoughts or outside advice, may have advantages from the police standpoint, too much is neither humane, therapeutic, nor fruitful.

Because a rapist frequently becomes a murderer, the case must be reported to the police for the protection of others. This is particularly important where there have been several cases in one neighborhood or where suspicious characters who loiter around children have attracted attention. At the same time the physician will want to take what steps he can to keep neighborhood excitement and police activity from blowing the whole situation up beyond what is necessary, thus perpetuating the unhappy emotional consequences for the child and for all.

Freud discovered in the early years of his career that in the course of treating emotionally disturbed young women they often charged that during childhood their fathers had approached them sexually. At first he took these charges entirely at face value. Only later did he begin to realize to his chagrin, how often the charge was pure fantasy. Yet his error actually led to an epoch-making discovery. He found that when a child or young woman *imagines* that she has been seduced, it may result in the same feeling of guilt and other psychic disturbances as when the assault has actually occurred. The fantasy indeed represents an unconscious *wish*. As a result of this conclusion he constructed his theory of the Oedipus Complex.

In addition to such cases of fantasied seduction or rape, many such charges brought against men arise from conscious malice on the girl's part; or, the man's approaches are the result of direct provocation. Often there is no sharp line between conscious malingering and hysterical fantasies; the patient half believes her own untruths. Though the cases which follow present a real contrast, it must not be assumed that rape cases are always this clear-cut. Yet even when one is fact and another fantasy, the personal and social implications of both remain matters of concern for the individual, for society or both.

Case 1 — Karen A., age 10 years.

Admitted to hospital because of rape.
Family Background: Scandinavian descent, Roman Catholic Converts. Father—employed as engineer; Mother—housewife.

Karen is the middle of 5 children with 2 older sisters (one married) and 2 younger brothers.

The Story—(from parents, police, neighbors). The family lives in an apartment house with a large play area in the rear, which is approached by a tunnel from the house. About 4 p.m., while the mother was out, Karen en route to the playground was accosted in this tunnel by a middle-aged man who talked to her, offered her candy, then grabbed her and pushed her into an adjacent basement room. He covered her mouth to muffle her cries, tore off her underclothes, raped her and then ran out of the building.

Karen ran screaming into the playground and hysterically tried to describe what had happened to women neighbors who, with their children, soon gathered in large numbers, attracted by her screams. The women plied her with questions and some volunteered that she was permanently injured sexually and might never be able to marry.

One neighbor then called the police who arrived in a squad car, took her to the station to get what they could of her description of the man, then took her to the emergency clinic of the hospital.

When seen there, Karen was incoherent, breathing rapidly and noisily, seemed in a state of shock with excessive perspiration and pallor. Examination revealed some blood from the vagina and scratch marks on her arm. Attempts were made to reassure her that she was now safe, would be protected and could go home as soon as her mother came. But even then she still could not give much of a story.

When the mother arrived, she wanted to take Karen at once to the parish priest who had been informed of what had occurred and wished to see the child. First, however, she was taken back to the police station to see if she could identify her assailant from photographs in the rogue's gallery. She could not. Her mother then took her to the priest. He comforted her and told her she had committed no sin and would be all right. In the evening at home the child continued to be restless, weeping, terrified, unable to sleep. She was given seconal. The family declined the suggestion from the hospital that she return for interviews with the psychiatrist or social worker.

Follow Up. A report from the priest 1 month later described Karen as comforted, composed and happy. He was continuing to see her frequently.

Discussion. As for Karen one cannot be certain that the whole incident has blown over and been "forgotten." It is possible that she may develop psychic or psychosomatic symptoms later on as a result of this experience. Meanwhile since the family are devout Catholics, the priest with his power to absolve from guilt may be the most potent force for restoring this girl's equilibrium and convincing her that nothing has happened which makes her "bad" or different from other girls, or prevents marriage and motherhood. His saying that she is guiltless may well convince the child, her parents, and the neighbors more effectively than could a physician.

Ideally, one wishes that the priest and the doctor could work together to help the patient understand the meaning of this whole experience and to forestall any possible future consequences.

Case 2 — Sylvia G., age 15 years.

Admitted to hospital because of "rape."

Family Background: Step-father, semi-skilled factory worker, Negro.
Mother, housewife, Negro.
There is an older sister and a younger brother.
Members of an unusual Negro religious sect related to Judaism.

Medical and Social Background. This girl has long been a puzzle to the pediatric staff of the hospital. She is a diabetic—has been seen frequently in emergencies for crises involving insulin shock, coma and bouts of abdominal pain. The diabetic condition is usually out of control; but physical examinations and laboratory tests have failed to reveal any other pathology.

Sylvia's own father is an alcoholic; she has lived with her mother and step-father for several years, yet she has always refused to assume his name. Although she has told many stories of maltreatment at home, she also expresses affection for her step-father. Both she and her parents have rejected any plan for her to live elsewhere. Attempts to help the parents see a relationship between Sylvia's recurrent symptoms and events at home have usually produced antagonism and a belief on the parents' part that they were being accused of neglect.

Medical Findings. In the last admission to the emergency service, Sylvia arrived alone to bring charges of rape against her step-father. She could not, however, give a clear picture of what happened. On examination there was no genital injury. Both parents were faced with the girl's statement and denied that anything had happened. The step-father admitted that once, while in the auto with Sylvia on the seat next to him, he had put his arm around her and pulled her to him, but denied that this was intended as a sexual embrace.

Discussion. Case 1 seems a clear case of actual rape. Case 2 is probably largely a matter of fantasied rape. There may also be an admixture of conscious revenge toward a man who both attracted and angered this sexually well-developed girl. It seems doubtful that the embrace in the automobile was as wholly innocent as the man made out; it is probable that it fired the girl's imagination—and, one could conjecture, her hopes. Frustrated, she resorted to accusations.

Though these are speculations, the experienced interviewer will probably get a fairly accurate picture of the realities in such cases. Sylvia seemed more angry than incoherent and was not as genuinely unstrung as was Karen. Her account of what occurred was fragmentary and inconsistent; she depended largely on accusations. Bad family relationships, suspiciousness and in general a poor reality sense all-round make one unwilling to take any statements in this case at face value. The negative results of the vaginal examination confirm the feeling that there had been no actual rape.

It was to be hoped that Sylvia and her family would be seen by the clinic doctor and a social worker both for the purpose of keeping the diabetes under control and of helping this hysterical girl who was becoming a delinquent. Hope lies in someone's winning the family's confidence and leading them to accept guidance.

Preparation for Hospitalization

Mention has been made frequently in this book about the reactions of children to the stress of illness and separation from parents, particularly by hospitalization. The variety of emotional reactions which follow such experiences shows that the child attempts through many bodily systems to cope with his feelings and conflicts. The younger he is, the fewer techniques in his repertoire of reactivity. Nonetheless, what he has are as powerful as any he acquires later in life. As a baby he reacts the best he can by crying, by not eating, by soiling and defecating, bedwetting, and not sleeping. His mood may be one of passivity, lethargy, and frank depression. As the child grows older he is capable of talking out his fears, expressing his anger with words and acts of which he is conscious.

Hospitalization may evoke any of these reactions not only at the time, or soon thereafter, but as delayed responses days and weeks after the event. For example, a child may not show his fears, or express his sleep problem while in hospital; but after discharge, days or weeks later, they may break out in full force. The delay throws off the parent and the physician who cannot understand why he should react so violently, now that things are going well in his life.

Severe reactions may be prevented to some extent by properly preparing a child for hospitalization. Preparation is always a difficult matter because many factors are involved such as age, reason for hospitalization, personality of the parents, length of stay, rules and regulations of hospital, to name but some. It is easier to prepare an older child with whom one can reason. Where a child can understand, he should be told simply and truthfully why he is going to the hospital. An adolescent should be told directly by the doctor about the need of such care and enlist his cooperation by sharing with him as much as he seems ready for. Presumably he already knows what a hospital is like, hopefully because he has visited one, or at least has heard of one, when he was healthy; yet he may still be uninformed and concerned.

Circumstances, techniques, rules can be explained and he is able to respond with questions and expressions of feeling. Preparation is more successful if done by the parents who truthfully assure a child that they will keep contact with him, preferably by remaining with him in the hospital as much as possible, and that he will return to his home as soon as possible when he is well. Parents should learn in advance the hospital's rules and regulations about visiting, so that they are accurate in preparing the child for their visits. Children also usually want to know about the pain, operation or procedures, and care in general; and how this differs from their home routines. Sometimes parents are themselves ignorant of these matters so the pediatrician must take the lead in preparing both parent and child.

16

All told, the child of school age is more willing to cooperate and can accept his hospitalization better than the younger child who is puzzled and confused by everything that goes into his care within and outside the hospital. With a very young child or infant it is virtually impossible to prepare him with reasoned facts and verbal assurances. For this age child the only ways which will help him to cope are how he is handled, how he is treated in the hospital, and that he be permitted to have continuing contact with his mother.

Young children particularly should get the feeling that they are not being sent away because they have been bad, that they will never return. There are several good books on the market which are written for children, and tell what actually happens to a child when he goes into hospital and when he experiences such things as surgery.

There should be no pretense that the experience will be joyful, like a party. Although pain and anesthetics should not be discussed in detail, avoidance of talk about them is unwise. If there is to be pain and discomfort, it would probably be less disturbing for the child if he had some warning of it beforehand, can prepare himself for it by talking it out, fantasying about it, and playing it out in games. Mention has already been made (p. 58) of the value of such abreactive play in dealing with sleep disturbances.

It is not possible nor desirable to anticipate in talks with the child everything that might happen in the hospital such as injections, and other painful procedures. Mentioning these might cause unnecessary apprehension. If the child feels that his mother knows about hospital matters in general and will stand by him, he is reassured. Hospitalization is best presented to a child a day or so before the happening. If told too far in advance, it may produce undue anxiety. Similarly, treatments and laboratory tests are best described to him immediately before they take place, preferably by his mother but otherwise by the physician or nurse with whom he is most compatible. Whoever it is should know what he is talking about, and should reflect confidence and reassurance in his manner.

The child often tells us by his questions how much he want to know, and what concerns him. He may want a repetition of statements made, explanations rephrased. Hopefully these will be consistently truthful. The child should be spared hearing the consultation between parents and physician lest he be confused by the words used, by anxiety of the mother, or by the somber and serious tone of the physician.

It is reassuring to a child as he prepares to go to the hospital, to talk about his return, and even to get his room and play materials ready for that event. This is additional assurance that he will be coming home again. Permitting him to take a toy or other favorite object with him to the hospital provides satisfaction and comfort. It will give him a link with home and the feeling of love and care that exists there. Parents should be discouraged from substituting for the familiar an expensive plaything or something new. The physician and nurses should make sure that the cuddly or favorite toy brought to hospital is not lost.

When a parent is able to tell a physician and the nursing staff about his child's particular habits of falling asleep, awakening, eating and going to the toilet, and where the staff is able to provide him with care which takes into consideration such idiosyncrasies and habits, the child finds hospitalization less upsetting, and less uncomfortable. Where children come to hospital with a pacifier, it is best that they continue to have it. Removing it because it is displeasing to a nurse is poor reason; the loss may lead to whining and crying on the part of the child, and intensify the ruffled feelings of the nurse who already thinks the baby has been spoiled.

As has been mentioned before, babies and young children are best reassured by the presence of their mother in hospital for as long as appropriate to supply the needs of the child, and in keeping with the mother's personality and ability to be reassuring and not overly anxious herself. As a rule, it is beneficial to all parties concerned if there is separation for some periods during the day, particularly when the child is ministered to by the nurses or when procedures are carried out which produce apprehension in the mother. The child may cry for his mother at that time, but knowing that she is not far away, the thought will often reassure and quiet him. A mother should be told to expect such tearfulness and not to consider it psychologically traumatic.

Since a parent's concerns and anxiety, or on the other hand his self-confidence, are easily transmitted to the child, every effort should be made to promote positive feelings and remove those which may be deleterious. Group meetings of parents who have children in hospital, led by a social worker, psychiatrist, or pediatrician, enable parents to learn from and comfort each other as they share problems, concerns and medical successes. Where children are chronically sick, spend long periods of time in hospital, such group meetings are extremely beneficial. Together, these people are able to support each other even when the prognosis is poor. (For discussion of the conduct of such meetings see pages 186 to 189.)

What is reassuring to parents and children in hospital, is the continuity provided by the services of a few key people. When a parent and child know that they have a particular physician and *who he is;* when they know that they have one or two nurses and *who they are,* they gain support from having some responsible person(s) to help them through the ordeal. It is indispensable to know a central person(s) to whom they can go for help with their feelings as well as with their questions. For the young child it is supportive to know *who is* the person in charge, and that *somebody is* in command.

Whenever possible, every treatment or test done on the young child should be done in the presence of the mother. Where this is not possible for a variety of reasons, the child's nurse, who is known to him as his "special" nurse, should be a participant so that the child can depend on her for comforting and for extra security. Moving patients to new environments in a hospital is upsetting, even terrifying. Maintaining the same bed, in the same unit in the hospital, provides security of a sort. Occasionally children fear that their mothers will not find them in the new place in the hospital. For this reason, no child should be moved about without being told that his mother or special nurse will accompany him, or at least will be notified about where he is being taken.

For older children, substitutes for parents who cannot visit them may be by other relatives or friends, volunteers, nurses aides and other adults who come in to talk with, amuse and entertain them. But young children and toddlers may be confused by too many adults talking to them, or handling them for medical and other reasons. Where play activities are offered, these are best provided by full-time employees whose schedules permit continuity of relationships. Children's reactions to hospital procedures vary; some talk out their fears, others repress them; some rebel, others submit. Opportunities to play out and talk about their feelings may be provided by "play ladies"—child-care workers who combine knowledge about child behavior with skill in work (play) with children. Children often spontaneously sustain each other in their suffering and search for security, as when older ones look after the younger, play with, protect and console them.

The pediatrician is inclined to concern himself mostly with the medical, surgical and nursing care. Where he takes the time to investigate the nature of other contacts the child may have, where he is able to arrange good contacts with parents while the child is in hospital, and where he and his staff act humanly instead of as merely medical technicians, children and parents benefit in many ways.

Adoption

In a country where child welfare problems have become overwhelming, adoption serves to cope with but a minority of such problems. Nevertheless a considerable number of children are involved in adoption. According to the latest figures on legal adoptions compiled by the Children's Bureau of the Department of Health, Education and Welfare, there are at present almost two million adopted children under 18 years of age in the U.S. In 1964 and 1965 three-quarters of the children adopted were by non-relatives and more than 4 of every 5 adoptions involved children born out-of-wedlock. A marked development in the past decade and a half has been the steadily growing proportion of adoptions arranged by social agencies. Also, in states for which information was available, at least 82% of the adoptees were placed at under 1 year of age.

In modern society there is considerable complexity and social dimension to the question of adoption, as well as the continuation of particular myths, fantasy and prejudice. The most common is the social-psychologic prejudice that since most children available for adoption were born out-of-wedlock, they are "wild seed" and as such are slated to repeat the sins of their biological parents, especially when activated by their adolescent sex drives. Another variation of this irrational theme includes the fear that the adopted child is biologically or intellectually inferior. Although the statistics do indeed show a high and growing incidence of babies born out-of-wedlock it is more a comment on the declining or changing societal sexual mores than the "wild seed" fantasy. As is often true of social bias, it serves to cover up irrational attitudes and is not based on our most refined knowledge.

Realistically the most important influences by far on the outcome of an adoption are the adoptive parents' biologic or psychogenic reasons for infertility and their motives to adopt children. Assuming that the child is biologically normal and healthy, these motives and attitudes of the adoptive parents are the most crucial of all the factors involved in the success or failure of adoption. In the pre-adoption interview the pediatrician can become aware of the reasons for adoption and the background of these parents. The degree of apprehension and confidence will vary considerably. Certainly the motives of adoptive parents are personal and unique. They range from biologic deficits in wife or husband to temporary or permanent psychogenic obstacles to conception. If parents have been able to bear one child but have been unable to have subsequent children, they will at least have evidence of their own adequacy as compared to those parents who have never conceived a child and feel that adoption is positive evidence of their failure, but nevertheless an opportunity to modify it. There is sufficient literature about the psychological inferences of adoption to suggest that the practicing physician be wary of stereotypes, profiles or categorical formulations.

In his book "Shared Fate," H. David Kirk, Research Sociologist at McGill University, views adoption as an institutionalized social practice of helping certain unwanted children become safely attached to certain parents who are unable or unwilling to have children via their own biological capacities. The goal of adoption in our society is the protection of children through placing them in a family setting where they can develop fully and adequately, and avoid the damage of being raised in an institution or a debilitating social setting.

But adoption also serves the aims of adoptive parents by giving them a society-sanctioned opportunity to have children and also some protection against having a defective child. Hence the adoption should be one of mutual benefit. Hopefully the child will find love, trust and confidence in the adult caretakers while the parents expect to find satisfaction, fulfillment and permanence in this relationship.

The influences of adoption are relatively harmonious when the process is adaptive and healthful. But there can also be dissonance or difficulties in adoption for psychic reasons. The disappointment suffered by a woman who cannot conceive and bear her own children is not automatically erased. The woman who has already made some psychologic adaptations to barrenness may also not readily abandon these defenses. As an adoptive mother she may be overwhelmed by the continuing demands and burdens of her newly-found motherhood. Just as the adoptive child may develop an identity crisis of "Who am I?" so too the adoptive parents may have to cope with psychologic struggle over the nurture of a child biologically not their own.

The physician can help the adoptive parents to join with their new child in a shared fate that promotes the mental health of the entire family. Although adoption is complicated by the fact that the child's biologic parents are replaced by his adoptive parents, the varieties of healthy or disturbed development stem from the same conflicts and forces that are seen in non-adoptive families. In fact, as a challenge that can be mastered, adoption like so many shared experiences can be the source of inner strength and richness. Just as a prenatal interview is advantageous in the usual pregnancy and preparation for a new child, the pre-adoption contact enables the physician and parents to know each other and to have the beginning of an alliance which will promote the effectiveness of their joint future efforts. In the pre-adoption interview the physician will learn something about the prospective parents' own childhood, how they were raised and what contact they had with other children, including baby sitting and mother's helper experiences. The attitudes of the grandparents toward adoption may also indicate potential sources of conflict confronting the adoptive parents as well as potential sources of strength and support available to them.

Many of the fears and tests felt by adoptive parents are condensed in the question, "When should I tell my child he is adopted and how should I explain adoption to him?" The physician will want to ask the parents how they would feel comfortable in answering these questions themselves.

Advising parents to tell the child as soon as he can speak carries the risk that they will tell the child dutifully and uncomfortably, often explaining much more than the child can understand. Often this practice conveys to the adoptive parents that unlike other parents they are duty-bound to remind their son or daughter and themselves of a fact of origin which may confuse the young child and create awkwardness or resentment in the parents. They may further risk exaggerating the virtues and advantages of adoption to the point where truth and reality are distorted. On the other hand advising parents to wait until the child is school age when he can understand an explanation about adoption and when he has adequate evidence of belonging to the family (and they to him) carries the risk that he will find out about the adoption from someone other than his parents.

Actually, either of these patterns can serve to promote a strong and healthy family relationship providing that the parents are rearing the child in a manner that suits the child and the family. There is little risk and there are advantages in advising the parents to answer matter-of-factly their child's questions, such as "How was I born?" or "Where was I born?" or "How did you get me?" without going beyond the child's question or his capacity to understand. Answers might be given such as "Three weeks after you were born you were brought to me because I wanted a baby," or "You were born in a hospital in Providence and then I came to get you because I had been wanting a baby."

The fuller explanations of adoption are more appropriate and useful when the child is older, after 6 years of age, when he can understand, tolerate and enrich his development through integrating the feelings evoked by such awareness. Just as questions should be answered truthfully, they should be answered in terms of what the child wants to know, not in terms of what the parents feel like confessing or ventilating out of their painful or tense feelings about the adoption. Also, explanations and questions can be expected to come up at different times as the child grows and in terms of the developmental tasks he is facing or solving at that time.

Just as the younger child will emphasize his curiosity about how babies are "made" and what happened before they were babies, the older child will begin to wonder about his first set of parents and what has happened to them, as well as why they did not keep him. The adolescent will search for his future identity in terms of his fantasies about his biologic parents as well as through comparisons to his psychologically real parents, the adoptive father and mother. Actually, his fantasies about the biologic parents will usually stem from disguised impressions and wishes about the only parents he has ever known.

Assisting the parents to clarify their own fears, fantasies and attitudes toward themselves as adoptive parents will often suggest how they want to elaborate their explanation about adoption to their children at different phases of their development. Similarly, the physician's availability to the child at successive periods of development should encourage the discussion of adoption along lines that concern or interest the child, ranging from a clarification of biologic adequacy to the illumination that the real shared life in the past, present and future is with the parents who have nurtured and raised him, not with those who were unable to raise him after bearing him. The common fear of the young adopted child that once rejected he can be abandoned again, can be reduced and resolved if the child is helped to discuss his concerns with parents who are prepared to listen and to reassure calmly. If the parents find it uncomfortable to discuss this fear they can arrange for the doctor to hear about the fears in order that he can explain to the child that the tie between the adopted child and his parents is as binding as that between the child and his parents who had a beginning biologic tie.

Common Problems in Adoption

1. The resentment felt by adoptive parents that their "rescue" of the abandoned child does not result in a miraculous fulfillment. They fear that if the child is not a genius, he must be ordinary or defective.

2. The parents who feel alienated from their child after they dutifully and with an altered sense of obligation explain the adoption as a lecturer or book has instructed them. Since the psychologic meaning of explaining adoption may be complex and highly charged for the parents and the child, planning, and preparation for the explanation should be unhurried and make sense to the parents.

3. The undesirable impact of the parents' "knowing" about the adoptive child's biologic parents and the reasons given that the child was released for adoption can be minimized. Enabling the parents to discuss their "knowledge" and their feelings about the "facts" can clarify and reduce a large spectrum of painful and disruptive reactions ranging from guilt to a fearful sense of uncertainty and lack of confidence about the adoption.

4. The plan to bolster a weak or conflicted marriage by adopting a child is often detected. Unfortunately, this may also become evident when a tenuous marital relationship becomes overwhelmingly stressed by adopting a child, which often leads to separation and divorce.

5. Often there is evidence of the guilt-ladened depressive reactions of a mother who views adoption as an illicit activity since her inability to conceive is experienced as the "will of God" or as evidence that she is an evil woman.

In each of these problems the physician through his sensitivity and awareness can become aware of the degree to which his counselling can minimize or prevent the full development of such difficulties and their elaboration. In many instances it will become clear that the doctor's care of the child and guidance of the parents will not be sufficient, and a referral for social work or psychiatric assistance should be tactfully arranged.

The pediatrician who is interested and involved in the care of adopted children also will be able to contribute to his own knowledge and to his community through close working relationships with the social and mental health agencies in his region that provide adoption services.

Fatal and Incurable Illness

The physician who decides to specialize in the care of children often is motivated by his fascination with vigorous, colorful and changing characteristics of the developing child. In the care of a chronically or fatally ill child, he may be confronted with what he expected to avoid by electing to become a pediatrician, namely death, chronic physical illness and the end of a life rather than the beginning of one. Usually the child who is chronically ill or dying will indicate rather clearly his fear of pain, his disappointment in not feeling well and his resentment and anxiety when he faces the threat of separation implied by hospital care and the course of his illness. The sense of helplessness experienced by a chronically ill or dying child often represents a composite feeling caused by the effects of the physical illness and its treatment, as well as by the impact of the anticipatory mourning reactions and depressed expectations of the parents and medical and nursing staff involved in his care.

The pediatrician in facing these issues in the care of a particular child and his family is confronted by a growing and somewhat contradictory literature. The apparent contradictions reflect the tendency of individual reports to categorize the recommendations of how to conduct the psychologic care of such patients and their families rather than to particularize the psychologic treatment according to the tolerances and capacities of child and family. Our knowledge indicates critical guidelines available to the pediatrician which he can adapt to the individual situation.

The parents and other members of the family will often react with anticipatory mourning reactions, which represent their preparation for the inevitable loss to themselves and their family. Mourning is the repetitive and intense review in feelings and thoughts of past and present relationships to the child, accompanied by bitter and resentful emotional reactions to the tragedy of a child dying before his life has unfolded. Such reactions refer not only to the loss of the child, but to the impact of this loss on family relationships and atmosphere. For many parents the death of the child represents a permanent severing of one line to immortality.

Since the individual's earliest survival emerges from a close physical and psychologic tie to specific adults, the painful disruption of this continuity by death or its threat at any time evokes feelings of catastrophic helplessness. This sense of helplessness persists beyond childhood even though the threat of such human losses in later life need no longer threaten the physical survival of the individual. Since the social and psychologic functioning of the human being is developed on the foundation of close personal bonds, the loss of a human love object is usually experienced as a depletion of the psychologic and emotional capacities necessary for the continuing demands of life.

The child who is dying, depending on his age and the nature of his illness and its treatment, usually selectively denies his sense of the death process. He may sense his fatal illness through the combination of his physical feelings and the perception of the grieving moods and the sadness of his parents and others who care for him (including physicians, nurses and others). The child may feel sad and frightened without being able to account for his reactions. If the patient is a young child under 4 years of age, only the closeness of his mother and father and the absence or reduction of pain will relieve him. Since intolerable tension for the younger child is often expressed through restlessness and motor discharge, his anxiety may be expressed through activity. If the child is over 6 years of age, he can find additional relief by having his questions answered in an appropriate and tactful way.

For example, 6-year-old Cynthia was fatally ill with a fulminating malignancy which seemed to cause little somatic pain. However, she was persistent in asking what her illness was and when would she be over it. She resented the repeated examinations and medical treatment until her pediatrician explained to her that there was a growth in her tummy that he was trying to help her overcome. He further explained that the examinations and medicines were to make her feel better. She said that she had been afraid that her tummy would hurt her. She was glad that the doctor would not let it hurt her too much. Thereafter, she appeared more relaxed, perhaps resigned, and less fearful.

In older children the closeness to death may be accompanied by anxiety, sadness and a sense of helplessness. The latter is particularly depressing in a school-aged child or young adolescent who has experienced the satisfactions of independent strivings and the achievement of social and intellectual competence. Anxiety, sadness and the fearsome sense of helplessness can be relieved by appropriate opportunities for the patient to talk about and understand what he senses up to the point of his own tolerances.

The physician who is responsible for the care of the dying or chronically (incurably) ill child is in the most advantageous relationship to the child, his parents and siblings to accept their fears and resentments, to provide explanations and to help them prepare for what lies ahead. In the case of the defective or incurably chronically-ill child, the parents must accept and adapt to a handicapped or defective one. In the instance of the fatally ill child, the anticipatory grieving reactions are a preparation for the devastating loss of the beloved child.

In relieving pain with analgesics and sedatives, in reducing the fears of loneliness through living-in arrangements or a liberal visiting schedule and in providing an opportunity for the child and his parents to talk to and question him, the physician has extended his knowledge in a therapeutic manner. Of course, where he can answer the questions of the child and his parents, tactfully matching the tenor of the questions and the tolerances of all concerned, the doctor can bring symptomatic relief by mitigating the painful fear of the unknown.

Denial of painful sensations, somatic and emotional, and of the knowledge of what lies ahead is often a necessary and effective device for coping with the fear of dying. However, this does not imply that the physician should encourage denial unnecessarily to the point where the patient and his family, who would feel strengthened by knowing, gain the impression that they are out of order or lacking in judgment if they ask questions or in some other way indicate that they want to understand what is happening. The doctor can be most helpful to a particular child and his parents by gauging their tolerances and preferences, as well as by understanding the significance of the customs and social values transmitted to them by their cultural and religious beliefs.

There are many levels and kinds of truth that are ethically sound and medically correct in meeting the questions and anxiety of the patient and his family. The physician listens carefully to the patient and his parents and observes what their behavior communicates in order to use that level of concept and explanation that provides relief and support. One cannot advise that all leukemic children should be told they have a fatal illness, or that no child with leukemia should be told what is wrong with him. A young child may suffer more from the painful fear of being alone (psychic pain) than from the pain caused by metastases (somatic pain). Both are components of pain that are indivisible.

The child with a fatal illness may suffer significantly from the adult's prohibitions against asking and telling about the illness. Children have often indicated, "I'm not supposed to know." Many, perhaps most children, cannot bear knowing about their fatal illness and its consequences; however, they also cannot tolerate a complete denial of the illness and its treatment. Depending on their age and the illness, most children benefit from explanations about what is being done to them and why. They are relieved by being told directly that they will be given medicine for pain and will not be left alone for long. The age and past experiences of the child and his family, and the conditions of human life in that particular environment, are critical guides for the physician on how to listen and talk to the dying child and his family.

The physician, the nurse and the social worker have the same responsibilities to an individual who is dying as they have to the patient who is expected to live. These responsibilities include relieving somatic and psychologic pain, familiarizing the patient with his own resources, and helping him to find and derive benefit from medical resources. The dying patient's resources that are challenged include the capacity to tolerate pain and to accept comfort, to live with sadness, and to review and experience crucial human ties as a preparation for giving them up. Knowledge of the illness, its treatment and what lies ahead may be a source of strength for certain patients and their families.

Thus, the physician's responsibilities and capabilities include therapy for those who are dying as well as with those who survive. His ministrations to the dying child can be helpful if they are not mechanically executed like writing a prescription. By augmenting his own clinical knowledge, and understanding, the physician can develop medical competence and effectiveness in helping patients face the fact of their dying.

As a protector of the child's health and development, the doctor can also provide crucial assistance to children and their families when a member of the family, especially a parent, dies. Through standing by, offering opportunities for questioning and expressions of sorrow, fear and resentment the physician provides one of the main supports for the bereaved in our society. The influence of the past, especially a death in the family, can be inappropriate and disproportionate or it can provide a perspective that is strengthening and supportive. Mourning for those who have died is appropriate and necesary. When mourning and understanding what has happened are significantly limited or not available, the past may live on in the present in attitudes, moods and restrictions that are inappropriate and that may stunt a child's capacity to form emotional and intellectual development.

A certain pediatrician who was keenly interested in such matters was making a house call on a bleak November day when his car radio program was interrupted by the news of the tragic death of a young lineman who had been electrocuted accidentally. The lineman was the father of three children who were patients of the physician. After completing his house call, the doctor proceeded to the home of the bereft family where he quietly expressed his sympathy to the wife and asked if he could be helpful. She tearfully asked how to break the news to the children, and he agreed to stand by and help as she explained to the children what had happened. The 3-year-old boy sat on his mother's lap, tearfully telling her not to cry, alternately clinging and running about to bring his favorite toys into the room as though to distract everyone. The pediatrician played a simple game with him while the mother tried to answer the 6-year-old daughter's and 9-year-old son's questions. The daughter asked how it happened and without listening tearfully asked if they would have enough food and if they would have to move away from their nice house. The oldest child asked why it happened and listened carefully when the accidental aspect of the event was described. As the mother further explained that she did not know all of what had happened, the 9-year-old boy began to provide explanations, suggesting that his father was hurt but not dead and explaining away the finality of the death. The pediatrician helped the mother explain that there would be enough food, that the grandparents, neighbors and others like the doctor could help them and that when they found out more about what had happened to Daddy, they would explain it to the children.

After the acute phase of the numbing, overwhelming reactions to the father's death, the children had further opportunities to talk to and to question the pediatrician. It was clear several months later that the most important help for the children had, of course, been provided by the mother. She had been able to lean on her children's physician while she explained initially what had happened, continued with help to manage her household and family and had been enabled to express her grief without overwhelming the children. Relatives, friends and the pediatrician continued to stand by. The physician's guidance was available to the mother as each aspect of this tragic loss was encountered and reacted to by the children in the next few years. The acute and accidental characteristics of this death indicated to the pediatrician that the lack of preparation would have to be overcome gradually, with each member of the family approaching the complex event according to his developmental capacities and according to his individual relationship with the father and husband.

Divorce

Parents who consider divorce are usually aware that such action affects their children beyond the physical or environmental changes wrought by custody. They seek advice from the physician about appropriate ways of "breaking the news," or of preparing a youngster for new living arrangements, even as they go about asking help in winning custody. Some parents want advice about the timing of divorce, and even expect the doctor to decide for them whether to leave their spouse or "stick it out until the children are older."

As we mentioned earlier in the chapter on counselling, the physician is well-advised never to make a decision of that kind. Yet there is much that he can do with safety and usefulness.

He can act as a defender of the rights of children. He does this when he meets with both parents and their lawyers, and sometimes with a judge in chambers, to help plan custody which is flexible, which affords a child the opportunity to have a happy and positive relationship with two parents despite their separation. Custody which considers the wishes of the child, even though he is as young as 4 or 5 years of age, works out more satisfactorily for child and parents alike than a custody which legally arranges a rigid schedule that is as unrealistic as it is psychologically unsound.

The cause of harm is the *emotional* "divorce" that proceeds and follows the legal divorce. As long as a child knows that his parents love him and will continue to take care of him, then he can accept the fact that both no longer live with him. But such knowledge comes from contacts, from relationship with parents. Separation from a parent precludes it. He may miss a parent, may hope for the family to be united, and have many fantasies about what has been, and what could be. The family is the center of security for the child. When it breaks up, he is worried about what will happen to him. A small child often feels that he is to blame for the trouble between his parents. Frequently he feels abandoned by them, or that if one parent can leave him, there is little guarantee that the second parent will not do the same.

Certainly, the young child does not agree that a divorce is what would be best for him. Although a 5-year-old may fantasy the separation of his parents, his over-riding conscious preferences are for the parents to stay together. Despite the desirability of a divorce, therefore, the child will feel disappointed or resentful or frightened—or all three—where the bulwark of what he perceives as his safety and well-being is breaking up.

The pediatrician wonders what he can do to help parents so that their children's feelings of guilt and fear are minimized. *How and when should a parent tell a child?* Parents often understand that they will inflict pain on the child with the news, and so they first feel anxious, guilty, and afraid of his reactions. Many parents feel that if they intellectually explain, the child will understand. A physician will be guided, as will a parent, in what a child should be told by taking note of his age, and what it may be assumed he already knows or guesses. Also the nature of the relationship with his father and with his mother should help decide how to present plans for an impending divorce.

Many parents put off telling their child until just before legal proceedings are started. By that time, the child is usually well aware of what is going on. Such children are left to interpret for themselves what they see, hear and believe. They are intuitive, and often assess correctly what is happening; yet their immaturity makes them confused and leads to misunderstanding.

The physician, like the parent, should take the clues from the child about what to tell, how much and in what degree of detail. Parents should be truthful, but this does not mean going into detail about marital incompatibility, or the basic and intimate factors that led to separation. Most children could not understand these complex relationships. Some mothers are able to say honestly, "Your father and I can no longer live together happily, but that doesn't change the feelings we have for you. Even though we won't live together, we will both continue to love you and we will not stop being your parents." Some parents are able to anticipate the concern of the child about his share of blame in causing the divorce, by explaining that what happened between husband and wife had nothing to do with his acts; that he was no cause of their unhappiness. When parents do not know about the actual time or the details of divorce, they should truthfully acknowledge that they do not know. They can reassure the child by telling him that they will keep him informed and will take his wishes and his "rights" into consideration as far as possible.

Some children show no reaction to a crisis like divorce, and the parents are misled into thinking that they have adjusted well or are insensitive to such things. Actually such children frequently are denying the truth and are attempting not to face it. It is a usual defense against a painful realistic situation. If the parent(s) cannot manage to engage the child in "talking it out" the doctor, as an objective person, may be more successful. It is best to face the issue directly with such children, helping them to talk about what they have on their minds. Although answers to questions should be brief, the manner in dealing with a child should be patient and leisurely, lest he feel that there is disinterest or an attempt to brush aside the matter as something unimportant. One can bottle up a child by hastily or superficially dealing with a crisis like divorce.

Older children understand verbal explanations better than younger ones about what is planned, or why their parents have decided to separate. Older children can ask questions, can show feelings of anger, resentment, guilt, and even (rarely) of pleasure. Hence they are able to more or less work through the problems incidental to the parental acts. The younger child will have greater difficulty understanding, yet even the very youngest senses the feelings of parents and the changes impending in family life. They react to loss in the only way possible for them developmentally; by changes in behavior, often regressive; by somatic illness. The parent needs to communicate to them through the care he provides; non-verbal, attitudinal and personal; affectionate and sympathetic.

Despite the hardship brought on by divorce, a marriage which is filled with unhappiness and torment benefits no one. Keeping it going "for the sake of the children" usually shows faulty reasoning. It is a lesser evil to divorce than to live a life of hypocrisy. Then too, divorce does not automatically destroy children. With proper emotional support and the confirmation of parental security they can withstand many situational vicissitudes.

One of the commonest complications of a divorce is the continued fighting between the parents, especially that related to custody and visitation of the children. The pediatrician who is serving the best interests of the child, his patient, can often point out to divorced parents that it makes better sense to children when their divorced parents are able to resolve conflicts in a grown-up way. What distresses and confuses the child is the guilt and conflict of loyalty evoked by divorced parents who remain tied to each other by fighting over the children, and who by their behavior seem to insist that the child should ally himself with one parent against the other parent.

As he hears them out, the physician helps children to find answers to questions about divorce, to express feelings of resentment against parents, and to plan new ways of living. Many a child finds in the sex of the physician the man or woman he needs to be with and to talk to, even though such meetings are infrequent, brief and in a doctor's office. Some children try to seek such "a friend" by complaining of feeling sick. Or they write letters and send postcards to him. Fortunate is that child whose doctor responds by also sending a card at special times, or by telephoning a word of greeting. Lucky is the physician who finds pleasure in doing this; it is "therapeutic" for him as well as for the child. Through this ongoing relationship and communication the doctor can assist the child in understanding that his past feelings and wishes could no more separate his parents than his present ones can unite them. Further, in this same way the child can be helped as he grows up to realize that he can love and be loved by two parents who have ceased to love each other—may even dislike each other—without being a hypocritical or bad person himself.

Ideally, the best time for helping a child is when his parents first sense their incompatibility as husband and wife, and become aware of what this does to their relationships with each other and with their children. Emotional divorce always precedes legal divorce; and legal divorce does not always follow emotional divorce. When parents consult a physician early and give him a history of family trouble, he is in the best position to make suggestions which may improve parent-child relationships. Unfortunately however, prevention of family breakdown is less successful than is desired.

Although most children feel the effects of divorce for long periods of time, many compensate satisfactorily. It depends on the nature of the custody, and on the manner in which parents are able to reconstruct their own lives and still bring to the child what he needs from each of them.

Toxic Psychoses (Mental Symptoms)

We speak of delirium or toxic psychosis when there is a stress reaction connected with an interference with the metabolism of the cerebral cortex. An acute infection with high fever is one of the commonest causes, but trauma, hypoglycemia, neoplasms and drugs are also likely causes. Various characteristic mental symptoms result. These are reversible when the infection clears and this clearing is one of the determinants of the differential diagnosis.

The important characteristics of a toxic psychosis are deficits in the pattern of awareness and in intellectual capacity. Awareness may fluctuate from a confused state that indicates an incomplete appreciation to one which comes and goes, in which there is sometimes understanding and other times a lack of it. There may be deterioration of abstract thinking, memory and recall, learning, orientation, and in the use of motor skills. Where the patient has some slight awareness, or mixed awareness, his deficiency in intellectual ability is also stressful since he is painfully aware of his lessened ability to cope with his environment and his impulses.

The clinical picture then represents reactions to or defenses against psychopathologic infringements, as well as lessening of the higher controls of mental processes. It is important to remember that some persons react violently to relatively slight trauma, others weather even severe metabolic upheavals without impairment of mental equilibrium. This in itself tells something about a patient's previous state of emotional stability.

Careful analysis of the content of a delirium frequently gives clues as to premorbid fantasies and thought processes. For that reason, the content of every disoriented patient should not only be listened to, but should be recorded on his chart for detailed analysis as to its meaning and relationship to previous states of health. In the case of a child especially it may provide a new angle of approach to his problems and suggest ways to improve his general well-being.

Principles of Management

1. As far as possible, maintain the stability of the environment and reduce excessive stimulation. It must be constantly remembered that hospitalization in itself, for any patient, is a stressful experience.

2. Reinforce the patient's attempts to perceive correctly by giving him suitable explanations and statements about all procedures to which he is subjected. The altered psychic state of which all patients with a toxic delirium are aware to some extent, is in itself frightening. An adolescent even in his rational mind is easily frightened by the procedures of hospitalization which he experiences.

17

3. Avoid the conditions of care which would stimulate fantasy; for example, complete darkness, body stimulation, and stories.

4. Avoid use of any drugs which might interfere with the efforts of the patient and which because of idiosyncrasy or even natural reactions tend to produce disorientation or confusion. Relatives of patients should always be asked whether the patient has ever experienced any untoward results from medicines. If a disoriented patient requires sedation, it is better to use a simple pharmacologic agent like chloral hydrate or paraldehyde, especially to control motor excitement.

Case of Peter R., 15¾ years old. Toxic psychosis secondary to infection.

Presenting Complaint. Admitted to the hospital emergency clinic for lacerated left wrist, fever and delirium. A week before admission to the hospital Peter had fallen while carrying a milk bottle. It broke and cut the dorsum of his left wrist. Profuse bleeding was controlled by washing with peroxide and bandaging with a towel. Although the accident had occurred while his parents were at home, Peter avoided them and sought help from a neighbor, a young married man who was a special pal. Two days later the wound seemed to be healed enough for Peter to play football, but he awoke the next morning with much pain and fever. He had no appetite, drank a lot of water, complained of sore throat and diarrhea. Soon he vomited, had headache and abdominal pain. After 2 more days his wrist and hand were swollen and inflamed, he vomited and had chills and fever. At this point he was brought to the hospital.

Physical Examination. Besides the swelling, there was a puncture wound in the wrist discharging pus; there was red streaking up the arm and the lymph nodes of the axilla were enlarged. No recent exposure to a contagious disease was reported. Temperature was 99.5°F, pulse 80, respiration 20. The white blood count, 25,000 on admission, gradually fell to normal in the next few days but he remained disoriented and seemed acutely sick. A blood culture was negative; the pus, cultured from the wound, grew out beta Streptococcus and hemolytic Staphylococcus aureus. He was given penicillin intravenously, aspirin by mouth and Staphcillin intramuscularly. The hand was kept elevated and hot soaks applied. His temperature rose to 104°F, where it remained for 4 days.

Peter was continuously delirious with visual hallucinations and it proved extremely difficult to keep him in bed. He ripped off his dressings and the intravenous needle. In attempting to flee the room he jabbed his right arm through a pane of glass. Paraldehyde and chloral hydrate were given. At the height of his delirium the electroencephalogram was abnormal in a non-specific way. This period of acute delirium lasted 5 days and when he finally returned to good orientation for time, space and remote memory, he had no recall for events of the immediate past.

After a few more days he was discharged from the hospital, his cellulitis healed, and his psychologic well-being restored in the main. His parents had described him as a normal teenager who gave no trouble. It could now be assumed that there was no basic psychosis and that his mental state was, at least in part, caused by the infection.

However, the content of this boy's delirium was highly significant. He kept shouting that he was being chased by a gang of boys who wanted to beat him up, expose his genitals and were threatening to castrate him. These hallucinations were terribly real and violently terrifying and it was felt that an attempt should be made to explore real or imaginary events in this boy's life which might suggest a basis for such hallucinations. Accordingly, 2 weeks later, Peter and his parents were interviewed, first the parents and later the boy.

History. The boy's parents reported that for the past year and a half Peter had been unusually secretive and withdrawn, in marked contrast to his former outgoing self. He spent a great deal of time visiting with a neighbor, a young married man who was unemployed, given to bouts of alcoholism and disorderly behavior. The parents had deplored this relationship but any questions about it met with angry resentment from Peter and refusal to talk. For some time, the boy had insisted on having a light on in his room at night and he had had a bout of distressing nightmares in which he screamed and called for help.

Peter himself was reserved during the interview, shrugging off any suggestion that he might have any special fears or uncomfortable thoughts. When the conversation was brought around to inquiring what he enjoyed doing, what friends he had, Peter volunteered that he had a special friend and described the neighbor his parents had mentioned. He said he believed the man was mentally upset, that he, Peter, "only wants to help him," and he believes his friendship has meant much to this man. Further than this he did not go, and it was felt unwise to probe.

Discussion. With this patient the history was revealing in that there had been no premonitory signs of physical or emotional illness, and that all was well as judged from the statements of the family. However, one clue that suggested some parental concern about the boy was expressed when the parents volunteered the statement that he was a good boy and had never given any trouble with the school officials or the police.

The setting in which the disorientation became manifest was in the hospital room, a strange and unfamiliar place at a time when he was acutely ill with high fever. The relatively sudden onset of his disorientation and the intensity of the signs made one think of an acute disturbance. The fact that the signs varied in intensity depending on whether it was nighttime or daytime and who was around also suggested that these environmental factors might be playing some role. The intermittent nature of the confusion seemed related also to the amount of toxicity the patient was experiencing, and possibly also the degree of his inner stress.

The diagnosis of the physical illness was clear-cut and typical of infection. The rapid clearing of both the physical symptoms and signs and the disturbed behavior suggested that this was a benign condition and that the physical and emotional conditions were related. The diagnosis of toxic psychosis secondary to infection was indicated.

The psychologic management of this boy in hospital seemed as important as his medical treatment. The former consisted of attempting to explain in understandable words where he was, why he was in the hospital, and why each step was taken, particularly any involving painful manipulation of the body. He was encouraged to ask questions and people familiar to him were kept at his bedside as much as possible. He was physically restrained in order to prevent a recurrence of injury by falling or attempting to run out of the hospital. However, the restraint was applied by people who spoke in friendly soft tones and tried to explain the reason for immobilizing him. Restraint was kept to that amount which did not make him feel uncomfortable but protected him.

Inasmuch as the chief ingredient of his psychosis was not only disorientation but anxiety and fearfulness, attempts were made to keep this to a minimum. After discharge from the hospital and interviews with the boy and his parents, an attempt was made to find other reasons for this boy's irrational behavior in the hospital. At the time of the hospitalization, both patient and parents were not suitable subjects for probing or looking deeply at any character or personality disorders.

Review will not be given here of the rationale for treating his infection, but focus will be more on the psychic manifestations of his illness. These may be viewed as a disintegration of the patient's ego functions and a breaking through of instinctual drives. This meant not only that the patient was unable to control his thoughts and his intelligence, but he was at the mercy of unconscious and instinctual forces. Because of the nature of his illness he had to be nursed. This further made for a reaction at a more infantile level. The strangeness of physical surroundings, the frequent body manipulations, especially painful measures, all added to this boy's confused mentality. Practical measures were attempted at helping the patient overcome the psychologic imbalance.

In assessing this boy's psychosis, not only did we attempt to determine the amount of anxiety, but also to interpret the content of his delusions. It will be remembered that this boy in his attempt to flee from the hospital believed that he was being chased by a group of boys who wanted to beat him up and castrate him. After discharge from the hospital, it seemed important to determine not only the state of his present physical and mental health, but determine basically whether there had been any mental abnormality present previously which had been exaggerated by the infection.

It was in such a post-discharge interview with the parents and the boy that it was determined that he had been fearful for quite some time, requesting that his light be on at night, and also explaining how he had been less communicative with his parents and much more confiding with a strange man in the neighborhood who was known to be himself psychologically deviant.

The fantasies in his hallucinations suggested that in his premorbid state this adolescent had been struggling with his aggressive and sexual drives, that he feared some kind of attack, possibly sexual. These impressions were not confided by the patient to his parents.

Plans were made for him to be followed in the pediatric clinic and there seemed to be no indication at the present time to refer him to a psychiatric clinic. Post-discharge visit to the hospital gave the boy and his parents a chance to talk about hospitalization and what had transpired there seemed helpful to all of them. Plans were made to have the patient see one physician, who was particularly interested and trained in the management of adolescents.

Case of Dan X., 14 years old. Toxic psychosis exacerbated by hospitalization.

Presenting Complaint. Dan X. was admitted to the hospital unexpectedly and precipitously without an opportunity for preparation. Ten days earlier he had jumped from a tree house, puncturing the skin of his right foot which caused him to limp. When the mother noticed this, she inquired about its cause, learned about the accident and suggested they not tell the father because he might tear down the tree house or blame the mother. The mother attributed some of the limping to attention getting. When he was unimproved on the tenth day, she decided to take him to a pediatrician for an anti-tetanus injection. On examination there was a puncture wound which obviously was infected, and x-ray films showed a fracture and osteomyelitis. Hospitalization was arranged. Both parents accompanied the boy to the hospital and promised that one or the other would remain with him constantly. However, the first night, after the boy was asleep, both parents left for home.

On each of four successive nights the boy awakened, confused and anxious, calling for his parents and demanding that they come or he would die. The resident staff urged him to go back to sleep, saying that neither parent was able to spend the night. During the day the boy angrily demanded that his parents stay but they refused. On the fifth night he had visual hallucinations in which he saw people walking on his body and trying to amputate his leg. The next morning he was sure that his body had changed and on the sixth night he refused to go to sleep because he thought that he would die.

Since the infection was not responding to care, it was felt that his condition required frequent taking of the temperature day and night, and much attention was given to dressing the wound by the nursing staff. The boy dozed lightly for two nights and on the seventh day was completely disoriented, had visual and auditory hallucinations, had to be restrained by jacket. His temperature was 103°F for several hours. The diagnosis of toxic psychosis and delirium was made.

The staff demanded that one parent be with the child constantly, that he be reassured by their words of encouragement as well as by their physical presence. This seemed to calm him so that he began to sleep for several hours at a time and on the eighth day, when his temperature was near normal, he was well oriented, quiet, not depressed, and willing to talk about how he had felt for the past several days. He was able to discuss his fears, the content of his dreams, resentment against his parents walking out on him, hostility against the medical and nursing staffs who seemed to be unnecessarily rough in administering drugs and other treatment. He claimed that one of the residents had scolded him and had appealed to his manliness instead of being sympathetic.

The mother's reaction was one of guilt for having lied about remaining with him in the hospital and for having pledged him to secrecy about the accident. She overcompensated in her attention to the child saying that "I would even brush his teeth for him if I could." She was observed spending much time rubbing his back, stroking his thighs, and giving more time than usual to helping him bathe himself. The boy was very guilty and conscience-stricken about his accident and the ensuing expense to his parents.

He became particularly close to one of the interns, calling him his only friend in the hospital and gradually confided to him concerns which he had long had about his health and the fear that he was not developing properly. He was confused about his sexual development, ashamed and bewildered about penis erections which he experienced when his mother and the nurses bathed him. He felt that he had been tricked into the hospital but was appreciative that now "one of the doctors is telling the truth about what's been going on in my body and what the hospital plans to do."

Discussion. Fear of body change is common in hospitalized patients who require restraint of the body or of certain parts such as when a cast is applied. Night terrors invariably appear after a few nights in the hospital. Even where nothing like a cast or restraint is involved, but after such seemingly ordinary procedures as a spinal tap, it is not unusual for an adolescent to have concerns about what is happening to the body by disease, by drug action or by surgical manipulation. Visual and auditory hallucinations are not rare after such operations. Often they are further induced by exhaustion when patients do not sleep well.

When physicians and nurses do not recognize the psychodynamics involved, they do not know how to deal with such patients prophylactically or therapeutically. Although the adolescent can tolerate separation from parents in hospital better than younger children, even he needs someone close at hand at night to whom he can express his fears, ask questions, and get reassurance. Grouping adolescents in the same room may be helpful in that each supports the other, and their mutual concerns are better dealt with. Such patients as Dan should be encouraged during the day to talk out what happens at night when they awaken. In nightmares they should be awakened, and encouraged to ventilate their feelings. Full recall may not be possible because it is not easily remembered.

During the day the adolescent, like the younger child, should also have a chance to talk about whatever is on his mind such as the cause of his illness, reasons for the disease or the accident, the plans of the surgeon, the diagnosis and predictions for the future. All adolescents are particularly concerned about their future and wonder how their illness or disability will interfere with their vocation, their schooling, their relationship to peers and even their marriage and having children. Giving of information which answers questions and reduces confusion also reduces anxiety and guilt so that it does not have to appear unconsciously at night and certainly not in the form of delirium or hallucinations.

The adolescent unlike the younger child does not need play therapy but the opportunity for "talking it out." He benefits also from listening to and from hearing professional persons as well as his parents give honest, accurate and factual explanations.

Acute Toxic Reactions to Drugs

As in adults, alarming mental symptoms may appear in children after receiving drugs administered as medications, or ingested inadvertently in poisoning.

The chief offenders are drugs which are used to depress or stimulate the central nervous system, analgesics, autonomic activators and blockers, heavy metals, hormones and the antimicrobials. The barbiturates, amphetamines, phenothiazines, caffeine, aspirin and alcohol head the list. Certain children exhibit alarming psychologic symptoms after receiving a drug which was correctly prescribed to induce quietness or sleep or to control convulsions. Yet what is considered an appropriate dosage may cause disturbances in those who are particularly susceptible. The sudden withdrawal of an anticonvulsant medication is not an infrequent cause of seizures, status epilepticus, or states of mental confusion. Of sufficient frequency to be alarming as a public health problem, is the ingestion by accident or with suicidal intent.

The most common signs of an acute toxic drug reaction are mental clouding, confusion, delirium, disorientation as to time and place, narrowing of fields of attention and of memory, hyperactivity. The child may be concerned with imaginary experiences, and there may be illusions, hallucinations which are mainly visual but in which all other senses may be involved.

The immediate problem is the management of the physical state, especially when life is in jeopardy, and control of the mental upset. There is need to control the patient so that he does not harm himself or harm others. Continuous presence of another person who can be comforting, reassuring, and at the same time able to provide control with humane restraint is indicated. Listening to the patient's distorted ideas and fears, without ridicule or prohibition of them is a safe approach. Answering questions accurately, persuasively pointing out the difference between what is imagined and what is real, helps the patient become oriented.

Drugs administered to counteract the physical restlessness or the disturbed mental state must be used carefully and discretely lest they compound the clinical picture with toxic reactions of their own. Paraldehyde administered gently by rectum and without unnecessary restraint often has a quieting effect on the overactive child. Regard must be given to the state of the body hydration, the feeding and nursing needs. The introduction of fluids by vein should be accompanied by words of explanation where children are old enough to comprehend. In younger patients, the presence at the bedside of a parent or another familiar adult will do more than words to comfort the anxious child.

As the mental symptoms begin to wane and disappear, a child

frequently wants to talk about his experience. He should be encouraged to do this within the limits that provide him with answers to his questions and explanations of what he has just gone through, and the reasons for his disorientation. The young child may prefer to play out his experiences and his feelings, particularly when he is not able to verbalize them.

Parents as well as physicians should take note of any untoward reactions a child has had to a drug and keep a record in order to prevent recurrences. Parents should be advised to report promptly any atypical behavior, unusual sluggishness or drowsiness as well as over-stimulation and disorientation whenever a new drug or an increased dosage of a formerly used drug is prescribed.

Psychologic Emergencies

Parents who seek medical help on a problem usually want prompt attention although there are really few conditions which are true psychologic emergencies. However, just as there are physical emergencies in the lives of children which require first-aid, so are there psychologic events demanding immediate assistance to the child, and frequently to the parents. In general, these are experiences which are sudden, more or less unexpected, and severe.

Typically such experiences involve the child who is disturbed by a traumatic sexual experience, a non-sexual criminal assault, death of a close relative or friend, learning about certain facts of life (like the first menstruation), sudden change of care (such as hospitalization), and new or extreme patterns of behavior in the self (as induced by drugs, fever, head injury).

1. *The Child Disturbed by Traumatic Sexual Experience.* A sexual experience is traumatic when it produces severe shock and tension within a child. Most common among these are rape or seduction, coercive homosexual activity, the witnessing of some forms of sexual exhibitionism. There need not be the completion of an act to upset a child; even an attempt at seduction, without rape, or a proposal of homosexual activity may cause panic. A child is frightened by the advance of an adult, and if his sexual feelings are aroused, as when his genitals are stimulated, he may not understand the queer tensions and feelings within himself, even if some part of this is pleasurable. The unfamiliar quality disturbs him. The child may be of school age and older, when normally there has been some successful repression of the sexual urges. Sexual arousal, even in assault, interferes with self-control and normal inhibition.

In exhibitionism, the older child often feels trapped since the event takes place in an isolated part of a building or community. The child feels alone and unprotected, may try to defend himself, and may or may not succeed in running away from the scene. An exhibitionist's display of his sexual organs, or any sexual activity such as impending actual rape, threatens the child's confidence in his own inner control. Afterwards he may, along with others who know about it, try to keep the episode secret, even denying to himself that something so frightening took place. On the other hand, the child may show symptoms which vary from hysteria to acute bodily discomfort such as pain. The parents and the community may be aroused to act. This action may worsen the child's reactions especially if parents and clergymen overconcern themselves with the potential for permanent damage physically and morally. In such an event, the child continues to have neurotic and even psychotic symptoms.

2. *The Child Who Has Been the Victim of Non-Sexual Criminal Assault.* The child who has been assaulted by a gang, a bully, or a disturbed adult (like a drunken parent) is surprised, because as a rule the attack was unprovoked. Such an assault may not seem severe to an outsider, but to the child it may be severe because of its relatedness to his own aggressivity. An older and hence more capably aggressive child tends to react to assault less with fear than with anger and hope for revenge. A younger and more passive child becomes anxious, even agitated. He may show prolonged and uncontrollable screaming, complain of pain (possibly exaggerated), which is first localized at the point of injury and then becomes general over the body. If there is actual physical damage, this may be disturbing not only because of the pain, but because of the body part which has been injured. Genitalia are favored sites for the inflicting of injury; they also are a main foci of one's concern. Apart from the immediate shock and fear of personal injury, there may be continued fear of "danger" in the community, disinclination to separate from home, and to meet new situations outside.

Sometimes adolescents meet assault with counter-aggression as when they gang up with their peers in order to get revenge. Police officers can be helpful by their use of protective and restraining force, and by the authority of their position. On the other hand, they may aggravate the situation by their own unrestrained use of force, and further provoke those who feel the need to fight their fellows. It is unwise for parents to criticize a child who has tried to protect himself aggressively, or to shame one who has been more passive in retaliation. A child will already be suffering from self-reproach. He may need help in developing better means of self-protection.

3. *The Child Disturbed by the Death of a Close Relative or Friend.* Not every child reacts the same way to death. Much depends on how he interprets the event and how it changes his life. This is related to his developmental phase and style, and to his past experiences. He may

grieve as do adults, cry profusely, and be overcome with feelings of helplessness. He may be aware of his loss of love and companionship with the deceased—or deny it all. He may fantasy and "solve" the problem in his own way by conscious and unconscious techniques. Rationalization is one. (See Chapter 6, page 97.)

Some children hold themselves partly or wholly responsible for what happened; or they may be apathetic and calm; giving the impression that there has been no effect whatever. Fears for health and life related to oneself or loved ones may be prominent. Death may be a shock to the older child's fantasies about his own magical omnipotence and his control over things that are disagreeable and dangerous. One must help him regain some of his lost ego stability. The role of adults is to help him realize that death, although inevitable, usually is not imminent.

It is sometimes difficult for parents and physicians to accept a child's unreasoning anger which may hold them responsible for the illness and death of a loved person. But this reaction is a projection of his own feeling of responsibility and guilt. The physician will do great service to the child if he discusses the projection for what it is, without attempting to justify his own position. A child who is not able to project somewhat continues to be guilty and holds himself at blame. As a consequence, behavior patterns persist which disturb him and his parents, particularly nightmares, protracted loss of appetite, fear of being left alone, failure to concentrate in school learning, and the development of various protective rituals.

First-aid requires attention to behavior which on the surface seems healthy, but which may actually be abnormal because it represents repression of emotions with later manifestations of psychologic and physical symptoms. The child who overcompensates with apathy and disinclination to discuss, needs encouragement to talk out and ask questions. In this the physician should as always involve other persons; particularly cherished, loved and trusted adults whether they be relatives, friends or clergymen. Such adults will also profit from advice on what to do to help the child, so that their efforts are productive rather than detrimental. The clergyman, like the physician, should be cautious not to increase the child's feelings of sadness, depression and guilt, but rather to reassure, encourage and make hopeful. After immediate emergency first-aid the physician needs to help the family plan the child's life and activities so that he does not feel exposed to constant danger from injury or loss of loved ones.

4. *Disturbance to a Child by Learning About Sex Function, Menstruation and Pregnancy.* Despite the advances in sex education for children, there are some girls who still find the first menstruation particularly upsetting. They do not easily comprehend the anatomy of their own genitals nor their physiology. They may react by attempting

to deny that they have had a period, discuss it with no one, fear the worst, and show acute signs of anxiety. This may be sleeplessness, complaints of being sick, taking to the bed because of weakness, nausea and vomiting, inability to eat. This kind of reaction is seen particularly in children who were encouraged to view their feminine role as unpleasant, unsatisfactory, and disadvantageous when compared to the masculine. It usually comes to the physician's attention when the parent is concerned by what seems like a physical illness of unclear etiology and unexplainable symptoms.

A physician may be fooled if he does not talk to the child alone, and if he does not observe her reaction to his physical examination. His suspicions should be particularly aroused if there is a predominance of vague and changing symptoms, and by the manner in which the child is reticent to talk about her body and its functions. The physician must not fall into the trap of making some vague physical diagnosis which will reinforce an adolescent girl's belief that she is sick, and that menstruation is an illness. Without lecturing on sex, the physician who can let the child know that he appreciates her worries and can reassure her of the normality of menstruation, will find a rapid therapeutic response.

Obviously, a follow-up series of sex education is also needed. This may be done to some extent by the physician, but he should discuss the advisability of this with the parents. They may ask him to help them make arrangements for attendance at some groups in church or in school where competent professional persons meet with adolescents to talk about all aspects of sex.

5. *The Child Disturbed by Sudden Changes.* There are many other experiences which because of their newness and strangeness evoke reactions in children which require special medical and psychologic attention. These include the sudden admission to hospital as after a physical injury or after the ingestion of drugs. The child is overwhelmed by the unfamiliarity of the hospital surroundings and the measures of medical management.

Surgery to a part of a body in which the child loses something, such as an arm or a leg, is as highly traumatic as for an adult. For example, some adolescents react with acute anxiety and depression when told that an operation will end their athletic careers.

Delirious states caused by medications, overdosage of drugs, or loss of consciousness by head injury comprise conditions which by the nature of the effects on the central nervous system provoke behavior which requires special management.

Children who experience their first seizure of epilepsy, or of diabetic coma, are frightened by the unexpectedness and severity. Some hospital procedures such as placement in a respirator, and a spinal tap, which are taken for granted by medical personnel, are frightening and confusing to a patient. Their reaction may take the form of panic states, delusions and hallucinations, overt anxiety, phobias, and anger outbursts. Some of these responses may not appear for some hours or days after the experience. For example, putting a child in a body cast often leads to acute night terrors 2 or 3 days after the child has been immobilized.

Signs, Symptoms and First Aid in Psychologic Shock and Trauma

Although growing children experience many crises in their lives, some represent greater psychologic traumas and produce symptoms which require first-aid. The elements which make this kind of crisis worse than any other are:

1. *The child's interpretation of the event.* It is of heightened or diminished intensity depending on his developmental phase and personality style. Children are developmentally more vulnerable at certain periods of their lives. Thus a pre-school child is naturally fearful, especially about separation from his parent, but he is overwhelmed with anxiety when it actually occurs, as when his mother goes into hospital to have a new baby. Or an adolescent girl who is confused about sex and fearful of her emerging sexual role may react to sexual exhibitionism of a strange man with greater emotional upheaval than the very young child. This is another way of saying that the *timing* of the experience is important.

2. *The child's understanding of his parents' feelings* about the matter. This triggers his own reaction. He is sensitized by what they have taught him and how they react to such things. For example, sex play between pre-school children is usually innocuous and normative; but the child whose parents consider this a perversion or evidence of a tendency to sexual promiscuity will be overwhelmed by shame and guilt because of their condemnatory attitude.

3. *The perpetuation and intensification of the psychologic wounds.* Ordinarily experiences which are psychologically upsetting are dealt with by conscious and by unconscious mechanisms; for example, by denial, forgetting, and substitution. This is an attempt at self-cure by the victim. But over-concern on the part of parents or other adults may unwittingly interfere in these attempts. The anxious adult does not permit the child to displace, deny or forget. Sometimes it is not the parent but others who prevent healing; as when police feel a need to question a child repeatedly, to have him recapitulate the experience, and to testify in a police station when adult assault is involved.

4. *As the culmination of a series of disturbing experiences.* Often one event in itself is not too unsettling and can be taken in stride. But when one event follows another, it becomes an avalanche of impact.

18

For example, children threatened or intimidated by schoolmates in high school "racial incidents" may continue life in an uneventful fashion and with a minimum amount of fear. But when the tempo of racial unrest is increased, when it is compounded by community riots and violence, children break down and require psychologic first-aid.

Evidence of shock may be immediate in the form of anxiety, hysterical weeping, screaming, excited talk, or extreme apathy. Motor restlessness, trembling and delirium are common, as is loss of consciousness, disorientation, trance-like spells, delusions and hallucinations. The bodily response also varies. Disturbances of the gastrointestinal tract (especially excessive or prolonged vomiting and severe diarrhea), and respiratory wheezing as in a severe asthmatic attack are not unusual.

After the acute manifestations, various chronic signs and symptoms appear, the most prominent being inability to sleep, night terrors, fear of leaving home or parent, compulsive behavior (particularly rituals, prayers, going to church), somatic complaints, enuresis and soiling.

Positive, prompt and rational first-aid can help an emotionally upset child to weather the crisis and prevent continued and avoidable damage. The object is to reduce as far as possible the tension within a child suffering from acute emotional disturbance.

Management

This depends on the age of the child, his symptoms and what is expected of the physician. First, it is important that someone take charge with self-confidence, assurance, and with the feeling of responsibility to minister to the child and to the other persons who are involved. Second, there needs to be a rapid evaluation of the patient and the circumstances surrounding his condition which will give clues to what next specific steps should be taken. Third, the child should be turned over to someone that he knows and with whom he feels safe, this being a parent whenever possible. The child should be removed to a safe, quiet, and familiar place where he can be held, cuddled, restrained if overactive, protected physically and given appropriate medical care.

First-aid should reassure the child about his personal security, and take care of his physical needs. Symptoms of hysteria, depression, suicide and physical illness require medical management. The physician must console, support, help quiet the child, without repressing his thoughts or his emotions. If a child exaggerates his feelings of pain, he should not be scolded. Giving attention to his immediate needs as well as his feelings of loss will reassure him and lessen his acute symptoms.

Questions which need to be asked should be put simply, and repeated only for clarity. There should be no pressing for details or probing to over-explain. The physician should sympathize and calm by his presence as well as by his words, but should not suppress the patient by appealing to his "grown-upness" or his assumed state of maturity.

Sedative drugs may be indicated but should not be used unless over-activity, restlessness and sleeplessness is extreme and prolonged. There is danger of using drugs indiscriminately with the development of side effects which add to the delirium, confusion or disorientation. If a child or parents tend to seek succor from prayer, by religious acts or in the expression of religious beliefs, they should be permitted and encouraged to do so. However, where a child or parent seems to express inappropriate and unwarranted guilt, the physician is correct in suggesting that while such feeling is understandable, in his opinion it is unwarranted. There should be no ridiculing or scolding of the child and no coercion to have him relive the experience. As time passes, there will be a tendency to repress, to deny and to forget.

This may have reparative effects and be to the good. However, if the denial and repression seem excessive, particularly when there is an accompaniment with new behavior which seems to be the product of the repression, it is best to have the traumatic event reexplored. This is usually best done in psychiatric hands, particularly to avoid the reappearance of psychologic shock which may follow the reassessment of such an important event.

One always looks in retrospect for ways in which the experience which led to the psychologic shock might have been prevented. This is not always possible, as when there has been a sexual assault, or when a parent has died. On the other hand, there are certain life happenings which may be anticipated such as menstruation, admission to hospital, surgical operations and others. Children prepared psychologically for these may well take them in their stride with a minimum of upheaval.

SUGGESTIONS FOR FURTHER READING

Abranson, H. A.: Psychosomatic group therapy with parents of children with intractable asthma. Psychosomatics 6:161, May–June, 1965.

Apley, John: A common denominator in the recurrent pains of childhood. Proc. Roy. Soc. Med., *51*, 1023–24, 1958.

Balint, Michael: *The Doctor, His Patient and the Illness.* London, Pitman Med. Pub. Co., 1964.

Brody, S.: Preventive intervention in current problems in early childhood. In: *Prevention of Mental Disorders in Children.* Ed. Caplan, G., pp. 168–191, New York, Basic Books, Inc., 1961.

Douvan, Eliz. and Adelson, Joseph: *The Adolescent Experience.* New York, John Wiley & Sons, 1966.

Engel, George L.: *Psychological Development in Health and Disease.* Philadelphia, W. B. Saunders Co., 1962.

Frank, Lawrence K.: *On the Importance of Infancy.* New York, Random House, 1966.

Freud, Anna: *The Ego and the Mechanisms of Defense.* New York, International University Press, 1946.
    The role of bodily illness in the mental life of children. Psa. S. Child, *17*:69–81, 1962.
    Normality and Pathology in Childhood. New York, International University Press, 1965.

Gesell, Arnold and Amatruda, Catherine S.: *Developmental Diagnosis.* New York, Paul B. Hoeber, Inc., 1947.

Grams, Armin: Parent education and the behavioral sciences. U.S. Children's Bureau publication No. 379, 1960, Wash., D.C.

Group for the Advancement of Psychiatry: Psychopathological disorders in childhood: theoretical considerations and a proposed classification. New York, Vol. 6, Report #62, 1966.

Hampton, P. J.: Group psychotherapy with parents. Amer. J. Orthopsych. 32:918, October, 1962.

Hoffman, Lois W. and Hoffman, Martin L. (ed.): *Review of Child Development Research.* Vol. 1, New York, Russell Sage Foundation, 1964.
    Review of Child Development Research. Vol. 2, New York, Russell Sage Foundation, 1966.

Kagan, Jerome and Moss, Howard A.: *Birth to Maturity.* New York, John Wiley & Sons, 1962.

Kardiner, Abram and Preble, Edward: *They Studied Man.* London, Secker and Worburg, 1961.

LeVay, M.: Concurrent treatment groups of mothers and children, Amer. J. Psychiat., *119*:1169, June 1963.

Lloyd, Charles W. (ed.): *Human Reproduction and Sexual Behavior.* Philadelphia, Lea & Febiger, 1964.

Lorand, S. and Schneer, H. I.: *Adolescents.* New York, Paul B. Hoeber, Inc., 1961.

258

MacKeith, Ronald and Sandler, Joseph: *Psychosomatic Aspects of Pediatrics.* London, Pergamon Press, 1961.

Maier, Henry W.: *Three Theories of Child Development.* New York, Harper & Row, 1965.

McNamara, M.: Helping children through their mothers. J. Child Psychol. Psychiat., 4:29, April, 1963.

Provence, Sally and Lipton, Rose: *Infants in Institutions.* New York, International University Press, Inc., 1962.

Richmond, J. B., Eddy, E. J., and Garrard, S. D.: The syndrome of fecal soiling and megacolon. Am. J. Orthopsychiat., 24:391–401, 1954.

Rochlin, Gregory: *Griefs and Discontents.* Boston, Little, Brown & Co., 1965.

Ryle, Anthony: *Neurosis in the Ordinary Family.* London, Tavistock-Lippincott, 1967.

Senn, Milton J. E.: Emotions and symptoms in pediatric practice. In Levine, S. Z. (ed.). Advanc. Pediat., 3, 69–89, 1948.

Senn, Milton J. E. and Hartford, Claire (ed.): *The Firstborn—Experiences of Eight American Families.* Boston, Harvard University Press (Commonwealth Fund), 1968.

Simpson, George: *People in Families.* New York, Meridian Books, 1966.

Solnit, Albert J. and Provence, Sally: *Modern Perspectives in Child Development.* New York, International University Press, 1963.

Thomas, Alexander; Chess, Stella; and Birch, Herbert G., *et al. Behavioral Individuality in Early Childhood.* New York, New York University Press, 1963.

Waelder, R.: The psychoanalytic theory of play, Psya. Quart., 2, 208–224, 1933.

Winnicott, D. W.: *The Family and Individual Development.* London, Tavistock Pub., 1965.

Index